REVIEWS for

DIY Ergonomics: Live Pain-Free and Save Money

"Irma is one of the most practical, fun and optimistic people I have worked with. Her academic knowledge and extensive experience as an Occupational Therapist make her the ideal author for a book on office ergonomics. DIY Ergonomics: Live Pain-Free and Save Money is an excellent resource and reads like you are having a friendly conversation with a wise and trusted advisor over tea. With Irma's sound advice, easy to understand recommendations and affordable solutions there are no excuses to not have good office ergonomics or to live and work in pain!"

Louise Taylor, Physiotherapist
Calgary, Alberta

"I've had the great luck of working with Irma in real life, so I know she's a pro at ergonomics. This book is a pure joy, a reminder of how to keep my body safe, and you can't go wrong with adorable stick figures. DIY Ergonomics is the most cost-effective investment you can make in your health."

Victoria Smith, Writer and Blogger
Calgary, Alberta

"This book is very informative for both new occupational therapy graduates as well as anyone wanting to increase their knowledge in ergonomics. The author is very knowledgeable and demonstrates how to create functional environments to prevent injuries in the home and at work."

Nushabah Zakir, Occupational Therapist
Vancouver, British Columbia

"I've been completing ergonomic assessments for over 15 years and Irma accomplishes something I didn't think possible – to teach computer related ergonomic risks and solutions in a format that even a child can understand. If this book was part of the public school reading curriculum, no doubt millions would be saved in the health care system."

Jason Dalton, Occupational Therapist
St. John's, Newfoundland

ACKNOWLEDGEMENTS

I want to thank everyone who supported my vision of writing an ergonomic book that would be informative, yet fun and easy to read. I received a lot of encouragement from friends and family – especially from my mom, Erna, who asked me "How is the book coming along?" every time I spoke to her and never doubted my ability to complete it.

I want to give a big thank you to Lori, Crystal and Steve for carefully reading every chapter and providing feedback on wording, content and those crazy stick figures. I also want to thank Kathy for giving up a weekend to help me with the book jacket – is there anything you can't do?

Finally, thank you to my husband for his unwavering support and patience; his belief in my projects means everything.

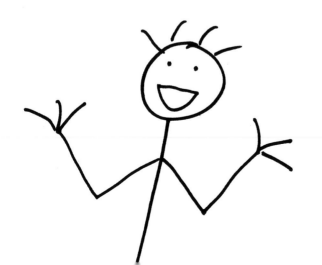

DIY Ergonomics:

Live Pain-Free and Save Money

written and illustrated by Irma Janzen

Copyright © 2017 by Irma Janzen.

All rights reserved. No part of this publication may be reproduced,
distributed or transmitted in any form or by any means, including
photocopying, recording, or other electronic or mechanical methods,
without the prior written permission of the publisher, except in the
case of brief quotations embodied in critical reviews and certain other
noncommercial uses permitted by copyright law. For permission requests,
write to the publisher, subject "Attention: Permissions Coordinator,"
at the website below.

Irma Janzen

www.janzenotservices.ca

Ordering Information:

Quantity sales. Special discounts are available on quantity
purchases by corporations, associations, and others.
For details, write to www.janzenotservices.ca

Book layout ©2017 Window Box Art & Design

DIY Ergonomics: Live Pain-Free and Save Money / Irma Janzen. – 1st ed.

ISBN 978-0-9958911-0-4

Dedicated to my mentors, Carie Lee and Lynn –
 for generously sharing your knowledge and experience.

TABLE OF CONTENTS

Introduction

Why read this book? Simple. I can teach you skills that will save money, reduce and even eliminate pain or prevent pain from occurring in the first place. This is not only vital information for you, but for your children, parents and friends!

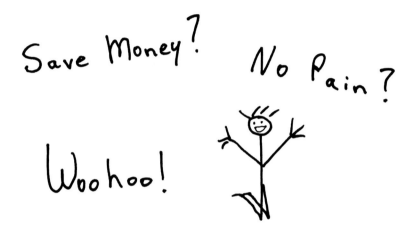

So who am I and why am I telling you this?

For starters, my name is Irma and I'm an occupational therapist with over 20 years of experience – many of them working in the field of ergonomics. If you want to learn more about me, I'll let you read for yourself on my website **www.janzenotservices.ca**. You're also welcome to send me your questions and comments through my email address, also available on my website.

I'm writing about ergonomics because I've worked with countless people who complain of discomfort and pain when working at the computer, or other electronic devices, who spend lots of money visiting health care practitioners weekly or monthly in hopes of feeling better and often get nothing but a short-term fix. Why? Because they haven't addressed the reason **why** they're feeling badly.

I'm puzzled by this phenomenon. If you stub your toe every morning, go to see someone to make your toe feel better, but then continue to stub your toe, why is it a mystery that your toe still hurts? Similarly, if you are sore from working or playing in an awkward position but don't change your position……see what I mean?

I'm not saying that you shouldn't seek help from a health care professional when you are feeling discomfort, but you should also address the source of your discomfort through an ergonomic evaluation. If the evaluation occurs early enough, your discomfort will often go away without the need to spend money on treatments for sore muscles and joints.

Maybe you don't know why you are feeling discomfort?

Chances are, if you're working on a computer, or any electronic device, your posture is contributing to and possibly causing your pain. Many people don't realize how easy it is to have poor posture, how harmful it can be to stay in the same position for hours at a time, or even what good posture looks like.

That's why I'm writing this book: to provide awareness, alert you to potential issues and provide easy solutions to make you feel better.

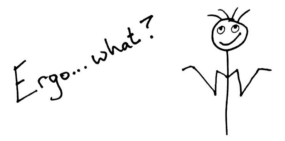

So what is **ergonomics** and why should ergonomics matter to you?

In a nutshell, ergonomics is the science of adapting the environment to suit the needs of the individual so that an activity may be completed safely and efficiently. For the purpose of this book, the activity is working on a computer, laptop, tablet, gaming system or Smart phone, and the individual is you or maybe even your friends and family.

It's almost impossible to avoid working with electronic devices and we need to be aware of the risks that come with these relatively sedentary activities. If you, or your children or anyone else in your family is uncomfortable or in pain and you think the problem might be related to spending time on the computer, or tablet, gaming or texting – why guess what the problem is when you can arm yourself with a little bit of ergonomic knowledge and know what the problem is?

This easy-to-use book is designed to help you evaluate your posture when using electronic devices – whether you are working in your business or home office, or searching the internet in your favourite chair. I will explain the basic principles of ergonomics, provide some helpful charts and give you plenty of affordable ideas for how you can improve your posture and adapt your environment when working on any electronic device.

Want a quick look before you begin reading? Check out these examples of good posture for you and your family on the next four pages.

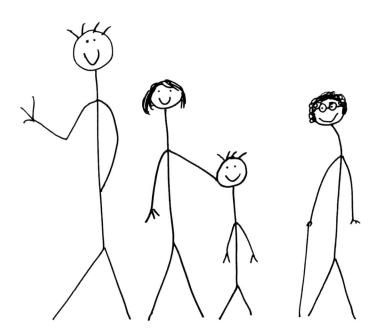

The four "family members" depicted in the following pages are using the same workstation but are able to adapt it to their unique body sizes by using cushions and foot stools.

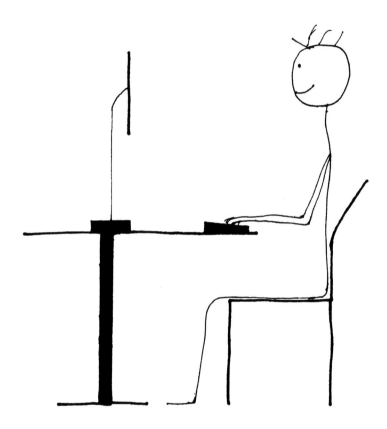

This **adult man** is lucky because he is able to sit at this workstation in a neutral posture without the use of additional props. If you are around 6' tall, this might be you!

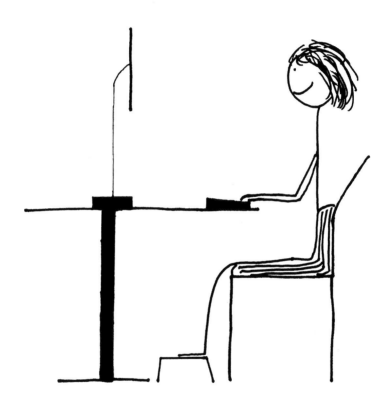

Smaller people, such as this **adult woman**, are able to use this computer workstation safely by adding a pillow to the seat and backrest of the chair as well as using a small footrest.

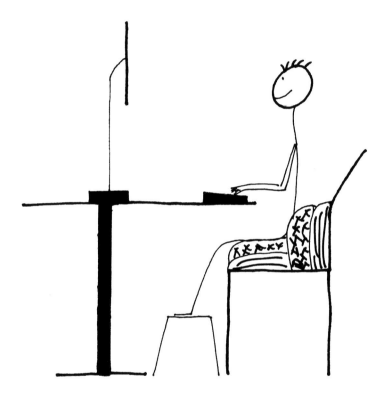

This **child** is using the computer safely and learning good habits by using extra pillows to make the seat higher and smaller. A taller foot stool helps his body to remain stable while his arms use the keyboard and mouse.

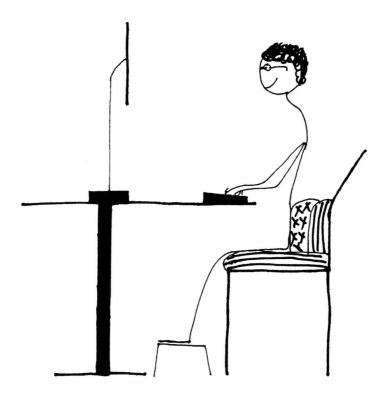

Older adults may have special needs when using the computer due to changes in their joints, muscles and eyesight. Decreasing the depth and raising the height of the seat, and providing a footrest allow this lady, who has a spinal deformity, to use this computer without aggravating existing aches and pains.

CHAPTER 1

Ergonomics 101 – Neutral Posture

If you learn one thing from this book, it should be this: Work in a neutral posture and get up and move once in a while. Bam! That's it. The secret formula for feeling good while you work at the computer. So the next logical question is "What is neutral posture?" So glad you asked!!

In a nutshell, neutral posture is relaxed posture. I'm not suggesting that you work on your latest power point presentation while reclined in your lazy boy – we still need to honor the spine and all of its naturally designed curves (more on that later), but we should also avoid overworking muscles and joints. Let me explain.

First, what's this about the spine and what's wrong with slouching in my favourite chair while I create my next newsletter?

> The secret formula for feeling good while you work at the computer?
>
> Work in a neutral posture and get up and move once in a while.

Think of the body, and specifically the skeleton and muscles as a machine – a brilliantly, designed machine. Our trunk is the core or base of our machine, like the foundation of a house, or better yet, the base of a crane. Our arms and legs are simply lever arms that attach to our trunk, like the arm of a crane.

If we saw a malfunction or anomaly in the base of the crane what would we expect to happen when trying to operate the crane arm? Breakdown, right? If the base of the machine isn't working properly, it is logical to predict that the lever arm functioning from it won't work correctly and might even break down and require repairs. And that, my friends, is pretty much what happens to our lever arms, shoulders, elbows, forearms, wrist, hands, thumbs and fingers when we don't sit properly at the computer – breakdown.

Of course, the body of our crane suffers from bad posture too. People are often baffled at the incidence of back and neck pain, but are completely unaware of how much their poor positioning is contributing or even causing the problem.

A great example of what our backs should look like when we're sitting is......(wait for it!) what our backs look like when we're standing. And let me get one thing straight. I'm not suggesting you sit in the perfect, upright posture every time your bottom hits a cushion. That's just not realistic, nor is it necessary.

You need and must sit properly when you expect to use your lever arms while you're sitting. The easiest example of this is working at the computer, but you can see how the principals of neutral posture can be applied to many activities completed in sitting, such as crafts, sewing, driving, among others.

Also, if you're moving a lot and only sitting for short periods of time, posture isn't as important because you're not staying in that same position long enough to typically strain your muscles and joints. Of course, if you have a pre-existing injury, any amount of time sitting incorrectly can hurt (if this is you, you're already nodding your head).

I'll give you an example. When my nephew was eight years old, he would start to watch television lying on his side on the couch, slowly slip head-first from the couch to the floor, pause there before gradually slumping to the carpet and before long jump up to grab a snack (or so he hoped). Non-neutral, awkward posture? Oh yeah!
But no problem because he's pretty much in a constant state of motion. The problem occurs when we choose a non-neutral posture and remain sedentary.

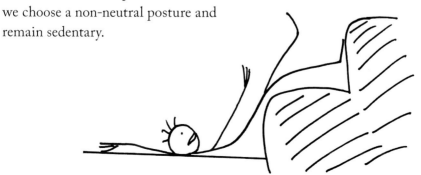

CHAPTER 2

A Breakdown of Neutral Posture

The Back and Neck

Our spine has several natural curves that allow our neck, trunk, arms and legs to move fluidly and with some pretty impressive range.

The only curve you really need to concern yourself with when attaining neutral posture is the curve in the lower back, or lumbar spine. Notice how it curves when you're standing? That curve in the small of your back is the key to everything. If you maintain that curve, you're golden; the base of the crane is intact and that crane arm can work as it was designed to do. Lose that curve and all the other curves in your back fall out of alignment and your lever arms just can't perform as they are meant to.

We don't usually "lose" the lower back curve when standing, but man is it easy to do when sitting!! Just a little bit of a slouch is all that is needed to flatten out that curve and cause the rest of our spine to move into an awkward position. Check out what happens to your shoulders and neck when you slouch.

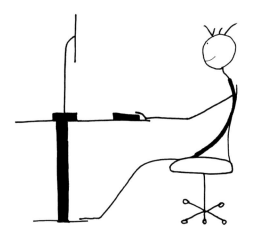 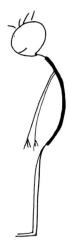

Notice how the upper body looks like a big, backwards "C"? Because the lower back curve is essentially gone, the neck and shoulders automatically move forward, which means that the head is also forward and probably tilted up if viewing a computer monitor. Because the back, neck and shoulders are in an awkward position the arms are automatically at a disadvantage. Their base is compromised – resulting in back and neck pain – and the arms are vulnerable to injury.

See how all of these risky, awkward postures can take place just by allowing that lower back curve to disappear?

Neutral neck posture means looking straight ahead without tilting your head to the side, or up and down. It sounds easy, but due to some common bad habits many people have difficulty maintaining a straight neck. This can lead to not only a sore neck and shoulders, but sometimes headaches as well.

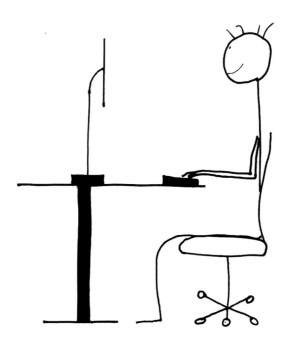

(Don't worry, I'm going to provide guidelines for how to achieve neutral posture in the next few chapters).

The Shoulders and Arms

Neutral posture for your shoulders and arms is pretty easy to achieve once you are sitting properly in your chair. Remember, neutral posture is a relaxed position. Notice the position of your arm from the shoulder to the elbow when you stand up and allow your arms to hang by your side – this is neutral posture for your upper arm.

If your upper arm is reaching forward or out to the side while operating the keyboard or mouse, your muscles are working too hard. If your shoulders are up around your ears in a tense position, or because your armrests are too high, your muscles are working too hard.

In the awkward picture in Figure 1A, the muscles on the front of the shoulder and chest are working to keep the arm in front of the body while the muscles in the back are straining to stabilize your shoulder joint.

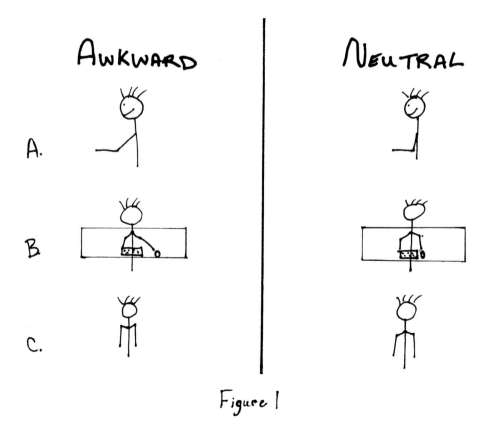

Figure 1

In the awkward picture in Figure 1B, you see a back view of a person working on a keyboard and mouse, and reaching out to the side to access the mouse. This position is very tough on the muscles of the upper back, neck and shoulder and is a common site of discomfort for computer users.

The third set of pictures, Figure 1C, shows the difference between tense and relaxed neck and shoulder muscles. This is a topic we'll discuss further in Chapter 5 when we look at armrests.

Many people don't realize how hard their muscles are working because they are resting some part of their arm or wrist on the desk or chair, but trust me, those muscles are working every minute that you are on that computer.

People are often surprised that the source of their neck and upper back pain is awkward arm posture, but they certainly feel the relief when they begin to work in a neutral posture. (By the way, I've created a handy chart on location of pain and the likely cause, along with solutions in Chapter 13).

The Elbows, Wrists and Fingers

So, what does neutral posture look like for your elbow, wrist and fingers?

Well, while you're keeping your upper arms relaxed at your sides, bend your elbows to approximately 90 degrees, and type or use the mouse without bending your wrists forward or back. When your wrists are in a straight, neutral position, your fingers will automatically bend slightly up to reach the keyboard and mouse. Sounds pretty simple, right? It is, although once you've created bad habits, it can be hard to break them.

The most common error in wrist positioning made by computer users is resting the base of the wrist on the desk while typing or using the mouse, as seen in the first two awkward pictures (Figure 2, A and B).

The resting position causes the wrists to bend up which is bad news for so many reasons. First, the part of your wrist that you're resting on is not designed to be a weight bearing surface. Go ahead and rub that part of your wrist. Feels a bit tender, right? You wouldn't invite anyone to slap or pinch that part of your wrist, would you? This is because beneath the skin on the underside of the wrist, is the carpal tunnel, which, when compressed or overused, can cause some nasty discomfort.

Second, the resting position causes the muscles in your forearm that bend your wrist up to work – A LOT. This can result in sore muscles and sometimes tennis elbow. Anytime your elbows are not bent at 90 degrees, chances are your wrist is also not in a neutral position, so watch that elbow.

Working with the wrists bent forward, as in the third awkward picture (Figure 2, C), can result in pain and discomfort too. This often happens when you are working on a surface that is too high, like a tall kitchen table. You reach up to access the table, but then reach down with your fingers and wrists to operate the keyboard and mouse. Again, this leads to sore forearms and sometimes golfers elbow. I'll tell you how to achieve neutral posture in your upper body in Chapter 5.

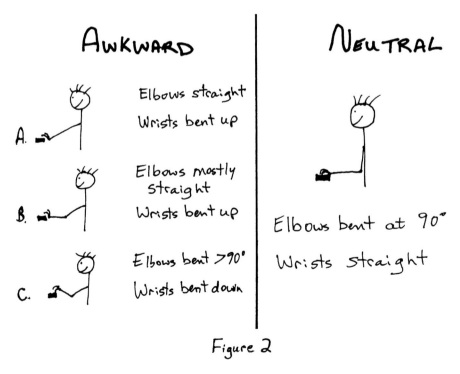

Figure 2

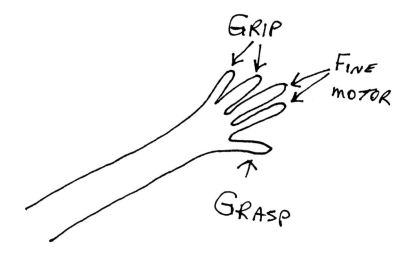

GRIP

FINE MOTOR

GRASP

The Thumbs

I've added a special section just for the thumbs not because of keyboard or mouse use, but because so often thumbs are used incorrectly and far too repetitively for texting and gaming.

The thumb is designed to grasp items; to work together with the fingers to hold something in place – sometimes delicately, as when you're writing, and sometimes with strength like when you're holding tightly to a jar or gripping a door handle.

The thumb is NOT designed to type, nor is it a good idea to use the same thumb motion repeatedly while operating a gaming control.

If you can't avoid repetitious movements, the key is taking breaks and allowing your muscles to rest. For fine motor work, like texting, don't use your thumb. Simple.

The body part that is designed to perform fine motor tasks is your index finger and sometimes your middle finger. The ring and little finger are designed to support the hand in grip strength. If, at this point, you are gaping at this book and wondering how the heck I expect you to text, do not fear. There is a simple solution which I will address in Chapter 7: Neutral Posture and Other Electronic Devices.

CHAPTER 3

Neutral Posture in Action

Applying the Principles of
Neutral Posture to your Workstation

Applying neutral posture while doing tasks, like computer work, can be tricky which is why I've broken it down for each piece of office equipment.

Don't worry if you don't have great office equipment, or if you're working at your kitchen table and chair. I will make several recommendations to improve posture and prevent discomfort that will include a range of equipment and budgets in Chapter 14.

Neutral Posture in Standing

As I mentioned earlier, neutral posture is almost effortless in standing, at least at first. After standing for more than a few minutes, most people tend to lean – which is usually a sign that it's time to either sit down or go for a walk. For those of you who still aren't sure if you're standing in a neutral posture, here's an easy way to check.

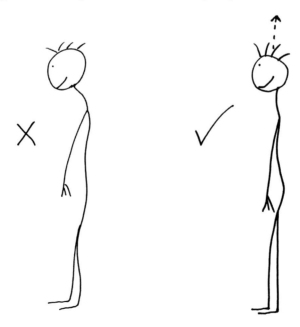

Stand tall with your arms relaxed at your sides, take a deep breath and relax your shoulders. Now imagine that there is an invisible string attached to the top of your head and it is gently pulling you up towards the ceiling.

This visualization always works for me and has helped a lot of my clients understand what standing in neutral posture actually feels like. If you can, ask someone to take a picture of you before and after the invisible thread visualization. Do you see a difference? Quite often, and due to bad posture habits, people stand "straight" but their necks and heads are bent forward. The "string" brings you back to the neutral posture humans are designed to have.

Neutral Posture in Sitting

It can be hard to notice when we're not sitting properly. Most of us are in the habit of flopping in a chair and not really thinking about our body or posture, but just on the task in front of us. We also automatically adjust our heads to view an object, like a monitor, so that we can view it properly, regardless of the position we're in. So we don't always notice that we're in an awkward posture because our body is so accommodating. At least it's accommodating for the short term; in the long term, our body protests, sometimes loudly.

Look at the pictures on the next two pages. In each, the figure is in a slouched position with the lower back curve either slightly or completely gone. Notice how the head and eyes are always in line to view the monitor?

FYI, babies and small children are fantastic examples of what great posture looks like. Compare their head and neck posture to that of some teenagers and adults - chances are if an individual has been using electronic devices for a number of years, they may be sitting, standing and even walking with their head bent forward.

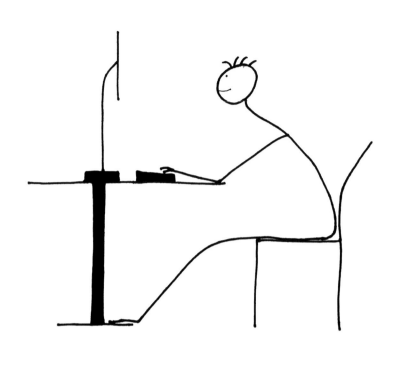

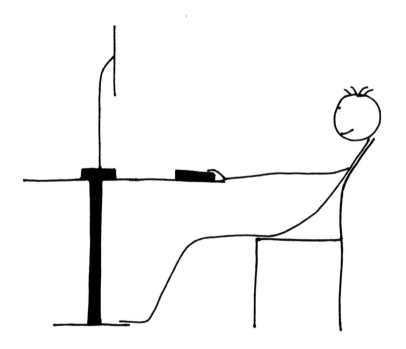

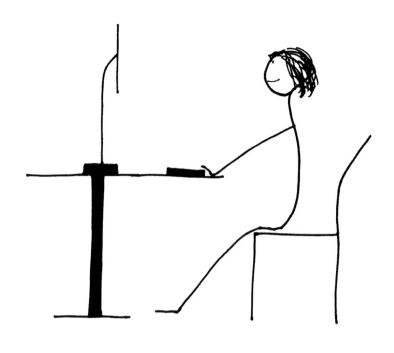

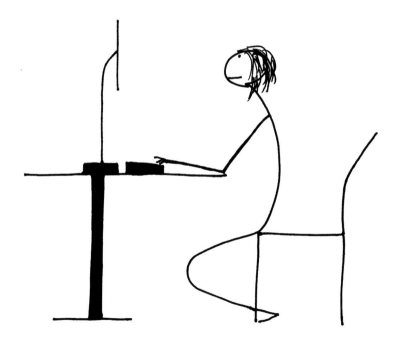

Some of these postures might even look okay, but let's freeze the seated back and neck position and see what it looks like in standing.

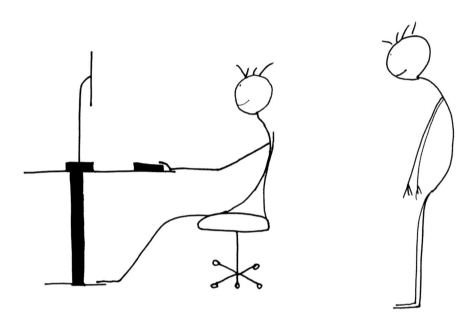

Pretty bad, right? Ever notice those people walking around with their heads bent forward? Take a look – especially if you're in an office building. These are people who usually look really comfortable in a seated "C" position, but once they stand, it's obvious how bad their posture is.

So, let's fix it.

CHAPTER 4

Neutral Posture and the Chair

It's not impossible to achieve neutral posture using a dining room chair, but it's much easier, especially if you're trying to accommodate several people of varying sizes, if you have a good office chair – and I strongly recommend you purchase one if you can.

As I explain how to achieve neutral posture in a seated position, you'll understand what an advantage having an adjustable chair really is!

When seated in neutral posture:

- Your bottom should be to the very back of the chair

- Your feet should be planted firmly on the floor

- You should be able to fit two to four fingers between the front of the seat and the back of your knees

- The lumbar support in the back rest should be filling and supporting that curve in your lower back

- The back rest should be tilted forward enough to support your back in an upright position

Keep in mind that most of us wouldn't question spending $1000 or more on a mattress, so why not spend $500 on a chair that you sit on for potentially eight hours each day? I've provided tips on buying an adjustable chair in Chapter 14 if you're interested.

Your bottom should be to the very back of the chair

And I mean **the back** of the chair. As in, your butt cheeks should be touching the back rest. This is how we should be sitting, people. If it feels strange, it will probably feel much better once the rest of the chair is set up. If it still feels weird, it might be because you're not used to sitting properly.

Your feet should be planted firmly on the floor

It's really important that your feet rest on a stable surface. When we sit, we should distribute our weight through our feet, thighs and buttocks. If your feet don't touch the floor, there's too much pressure on your bottom and thighs and it's uncomfortable at best. At worst, it can cause or worsen back pain and sciatica.

If you can't touch the floor with your feet, lower your chair; however if lowering the chair means you're too short to use the keyboard and mouse correctly, keep your chair up but use a foot rest to give your feet a surface to rest on.

You can use a footrest recommended in Chapter 14, but feel free to use any big book, foot stool or box that is handy. Just be careful not to raise your knees too high by using too large of a box. If you do this, you'll be in the same boat as tall people whose feet are definitely firmly on the floor, but whose knees are headed skywards.

If your knees are higher than your hips when you're sitting, you'll be just as uncomfortable as if your feet were dangling inches from the floor.

Again, this is because your weight is meant to be distributed between your feet, thighs and buttocks. If not enough of your thighs are resting on the chair, your weight is almost completely supported by your feet and buttocks, which tends to be uncomfortable.

To solve this problem, raise your chair and if necessary, raise the height of your table or desk to accommodate the new chair position. As a guideline, your hips and knees should be at about the same height or your hips slightly higher.

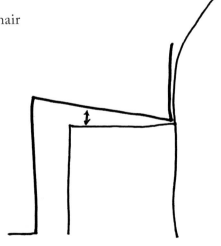

You should be able to fit two to four fingers between the front of the seat and the back of your knees

Sitting with your bottom at the back of the chair with less than one finger width between the seat and your knees will be either impossible or really uncomfortable. Many shorter people perch on the edge of their seats for this reason – it's just too uncomfortable to sit with the seat pressing into the back of your knees.

Unfortunately, perching means you're not able to take advantage of the support of the backrest, and I don't care how fit you are, you can't maintain that lower curve in your back for hours without support.

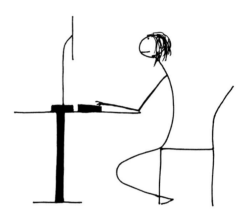

What if you're tall? Too much space between the back of your knees and the front of the chair is just as bad as having your knees higher than your hips – no thigh support, leading to anything from numb-bum to sore back and sciatica.

So what do tall people do to compensate? They look to support their body on any chair surface that is available, usually by slouching and reclining the backrest or leaning heavily on the armrests.

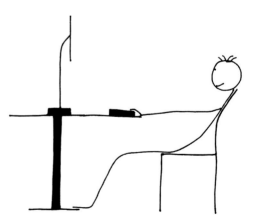

You can fix both of these problems by adjusting the chair's seat depth – yup, the seat depth. This is an important and often forgotten feature of the adjustable office chair. If you are between 5'4" and 6' tall, chances are you will fit a standard seat depth, but if you are taller or shorter, or sharing your chair with a taller or shorter person, it really pays to invest in a chair with adjustable seat depth.

If you are using a dining room chair, you can correct awkward positioning by being inventive with cushions. Place cushions in the back of the chair to adjust seat depth and use cushions on the seat to raise your sitting height.

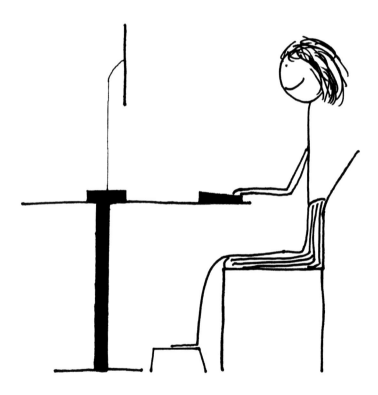

The lumbar support in the back rest should be filling and supporting that curve in your lower back

Lumbar support, as in support for that all important curve in the small of your back, is the goal of sitting properly.

- Do not buy an office chair unless it has lumbar support, or you may as well be sitting on an expensive crate.
- Do not buy an office chair that doesn't have *adjustable* lumbar support, because unless the chair was based on a model of your body, it won't fit you.

With your bottom at the very back of the chair, note if the lumbar support is filling the curve. Adjust the lumbar support up or down as needed – sometimes it takes a few tries to get it right. If the lumbar support is too low, it might be comfortable for an hour or so but eventually you will feel sore. If the lumbar support is too high, you'll feel like you are being pushed out of the chair.

Pillows and towels can be used to create lumbar support if you're using a dining room chair, but be prepared to readjust every time you get up. It can feel time consuming to spend a few moments adjusting your chair and pillows, but it is sooooo worth it to have healthy muscles and joints for the long term.

The back rest should be tilted forward enough to support your back in an upright position

Not all adjustable chairs have a back rest that has an incline/recline feature, but the good ones do. You will likely be surprised at how upright you should be sitting in order to duplicate your posture in standing.

Here's a trick I find helpful when determining how upright you should be sitting and how far to adjust your chair. Still sitting with your bottom to the back of the chair, sit up as if you are attending a basketball or hockey game and you're sitting on benches or bleachers with no back rest.

Okay, I know most of us slouch like crazy when we're sitting on seats with no back support, but every so often we all need to sit up and straighten our backs before we slump back down again. That straight back posture is where our back and spine want to be, and can be with the help of a good back rest.

Once you're in this position, adjust the chair so that it touches and supports your back. You may need to readjust the lumbar support and seat depth since you have moved your upper body forward. You will likely feel very upright, but most people find this position very supportive and comfortable, especially when actively typing or using a mouse.

You obviously don't have the option of adjusting the back rest on your dining room chair, but you can try to keep your pillows upright to create a similar effect.

Now, as I mentioned earlier, it's not realistic or necessary to sit following these instructions all the time, but when you expect your body and particularly your arms to work for you for hours at a time and for consecutive days, you need to set up the machine that is your body correctly to avoid breakdowns and costly repairs.

Also, sitting with perfect posture does not mean you will never feel sore or have a computer-related injury. You also need to move. I'll talk more about this in Chapter 8: Other Risk Factors for Computer Related Injuries. For now, just know that your body was designed to move.

When you can't move because you are expected to work on something that requires you to sit, you still need to get up and move periodically to avoid injury. Get up and walk around every time you start to feel tired or uncomfortable – a five minute break every hour is ideal and definitely take more frequent breaks if you have a history of injury or a health concern.

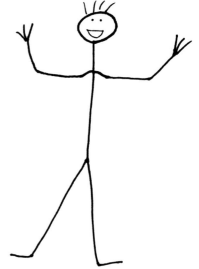

CHAPTER 5

Neutral Posture and the Keyboard & Mouse

At this point, you might be wondering if I've forgotten that the ultimate goal is to use the computer pain-free and not just to sit upright in a chair. Never fear, I've got you covered.

Although I haven't told you yet how to work at the computer with your arms, elbows, wrists and fingers in a neutral posture, the fact that you are sitting properly means that the majority of the work is done.

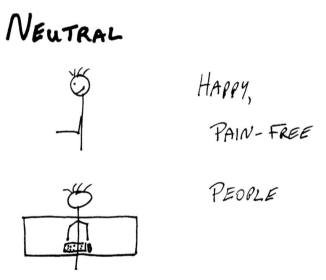

If you are sitting correctly, your upper arms should be resting comfortably at your sides – good! Keep them there. Remember, if your upper arms are reaching forward or to the side, your muscles are working too hard.

The key to using the keyboard and mouse in neutral posture is to sit close enough that you don't need to reach for these devices. If you're in the habit of sitting too far back, don't worry, you'll get used to the new posture and your neck, back and shoulders will thank you.

Neutral Posture and the Keyboard

So, with your upper arms in a relaxed, neutral posture, keep your elbows bent at about 90 degrees. You should be close enough to the keyboard that you can comfortably reach the keys.

Also, and this is very important, do not rest your wrists on the desk or table while you type. This a big no-no. Remember our conversation about the carpal tunnel in Chapter 2? The carpal tunnel is a very vulnerable structure and isn't designed to have weight put on it.

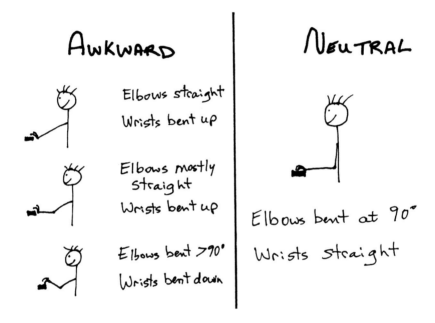

Basically, every time you rest the base of your wrist on a hard surface, you are squeezing all the important structures in your carpal tunnel, including blood vessels, tendons and a very sensitive nerve. This action won't cause immediate problems, but over time you can develop tingling and pain in your hands that is hard to get rid of.

So how do you avoid resting on your wrists? If you play the piano, chances are you have been taught to keep your wrists straight and free-floating while playing and this skill has automatically transitioned to the keyboard. If it hasn't, or if you're not a piano player, there are a few other ways to achieve this.

First, you can teach yourself to keep your wrists straight and floating above the keyboard – putting the keyboard at the edge of the desk helps. It can be really hard to break the habit of resting your wrists, so another tip is to put a piece of tape on your wrist when it's in a straight position. The piece of tape will pull on your skin when you try to bend your wrist, giving you a gentle reminder to keep your wrists straight.

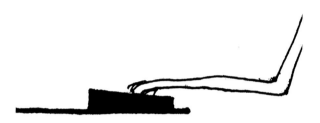

The second way you can keep your wrists straight while typing is by resting your forearms on the armrests of your chair – properly. I'm emphasizing the word "properly" because so many people misuse their armrests. Let me explain.

I didn't mention armrests when discussing the important features of sitting properly in your chair because I consider armrests to be....sort of the icing on the cake for chair parts, rather than an essential feature. The seat depth and height, and the lumbar support in the backrest are far more important features, and yet many people feel dependent on their armrests. This is probably because they are not seated properly and are simply looking for support wherever they can find it.

Using armrests improperly can lead to discomfort and pain, so how are armrests meant to be used?

Armrests should be:

- High enough that the forearm is supported comfortably, but not so high that your shoulders don't feel relaxed (Neutral Figure A).
- Positioned close to the body. If you're lucky and your chair has arms that pivot or move laterally, move the armrests inwards, directly under your shoulders. Now place your forearms on the armrests (Neutral Figure B).
- A support for your forearms, not your elbows. Putting weight through your elbows can result in nerve compression (Neutral Figures A & B).

Armrests should **not** be:

- So high that your shoulders are raised (Awkward Figure A).
- Positioned away from the body. This position does not support your arms for computer work, but encourages leaning, which contributes to back and shoulder pain (Awkward Figure B).
- A means of propping up your body in a seated position using your elbows or hands (Awkward Figures B & C).

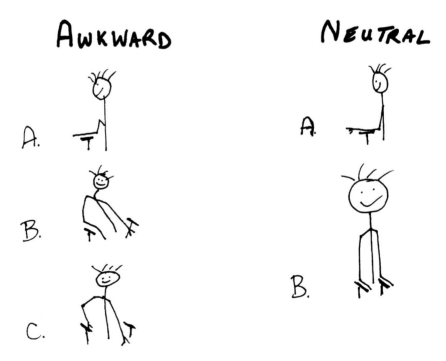

AWKWARD

A.

B.

C.

NEUTRAL

A.

B.

If these awkward positions look familiar, you are probably experiencing shoulder and back pain – including low back pain. Stop it! Your body doesn't like sitting this way. Set up your armrests properly and make a conscious decision not to lean or otherwise prop yourself up with your armrests. Consider improving your core strength so that the muscles of your torso, not the armrests of your chair, support your skeleton in a seated position.

Your armrests should support your neutral posture, not force your arm and shoulder into a muscle-fatiguing position.

Used properly, armrests will assist you to sit with your wrists positioned so that they have great access to the keyboard and mouse. Presto! You're relaxed, you're in a neutral posture and you're *not* crushing your carpal tunnel.

Neutral Posture and the Mouse

A lot of what we learned about neutral posture and the keyboard can be applied to the mouse as well.

You definitely do not want to rest the base of your wrist while using the mouse. Remember that this wrist position not only puts weight on the carpal tunnel, but results in the wrist being bent upward, which may actually lead to fatigue of the forearm muscles and even tennis elbow.

We'll talk more about typical sources of discomfort and their respective solutions in the chart located in Chapter 13.

I keep mentioning that the base of your wrist is not a weight bearing surface – so what is? If you watch how you do some of your daily tasks, you'll already have the answer.

When you push yourself off a chair, slap your hand enthusiastically on the table, or do a push-up you are using the parts of your hand that are designed to carry weight – namely, the side of your hand below your pinky finger and the area just below the thumb.

These are the meatiest part of our hands because they are designed to bear weight. Look at your hand the next time you use a pen or pencil; where do you rest your hand when holding a fork? You naturally rest your hand in one or both of those two areas of the palm, and that's where you should be resting your hand when using a mouse.

There are two different styles of mouse that I frequently recommend. The first is a vertical mouse, which requires you to rest on the pinky side of your hand while using the mouse. The second is any mouse that allows you to keep your hand palm down, as with a traditional mouse, BUT supports the hand so that the base of the wrist is not resting on the desk or table. (You can get more information on equipment in Chapter 14: Ergonomic Solutions for All Budgets).

It can take time to learn to operate a mouse with your hand in a new position, but I have heard people literally sigh with relief when finally using a mouse that doesn't hurt their wrists and forearms.

So far I've been focusing on neutral wrist posture when working with the mouse, but neutral shoulder and upper arm posture is equally important.

The usual culprit for awkward shoulder and arm posture when using the mouse is reaching too far for it. If the mouse is too far away, your upper arm can't remain relaxed at your side and you will automatically reach forward for the mouse. For the sake of your poor, hardworking shoulder and neck muscles, please bring the mouse closer and make sure you are sitting close enough to the keyboard and mouse to achieve neutral posture.

The other potential shoulder and upper arm issue is positioning the mouse too far to the side. This is such a common problem and so easily solved. Most times the reason the mouse is positioned so far to the side is because the keyboard is too wide. Solution? Get a narrower keyboard.

Of course, some computer users combine both of these awkward postures and reach forward AND to the side to access the mouse. I can't impress how important it is to keep the mouse close. I guarantee that

Awkward

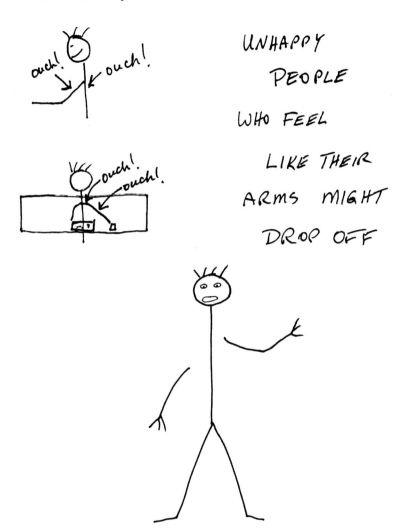

UNHAPPY PEOPLE WHO FEEL LIKE THEIR ARMS MIGHT DROP OFF

you use the mouse at least twice as much as the keyboard, and often more, so be mindful of where your mouse is located.

I know not everyone can afford brand new equipment, but sometimes buying a keyboard, mouse and even a chair is a wise investment and far more affordable that being injured.

Remember, Live Pain-Free and Save Money!

CHAPTER 6

Neutral Posture and Other Office Equipment

Neutral Posture and the Monitor

Most people position their monitor too high. Ideally, you want to sit up nice and tall, look straight ahead and see the top of the monitor screen. Here's why. Our relaxed forward gaze is about 15 to 30 degrees below what we see if we make a point of looking directly ahead, hence we typically see the top half of the screen effortlessly and tilt the head down slightly to view the bottom half.

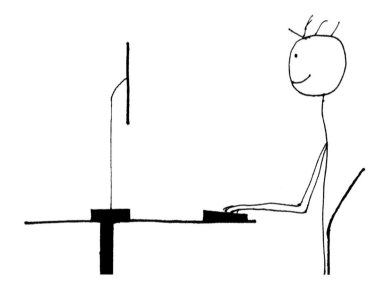

Biomechanically, looking up is harder on your neck than looking down, especially if you are not seated properly which usually means your shoulders and neck are bent forward. If you wear multi-lens or progressive glasses, you may need to play around with the height a bit, but aim for the position that allows you to see with the least amount of awkward posture.

The height of your monitor is not the only important factor when considering neutral posture and the monitor. You must also be careful to centre the monitor directly in front of you along with the keyboard and mouse.

I've painfully witnessed many computer users looking to the left or right to view their monitor. This very awkward posture is not only painful, but can lead to shortening of some of the neck muscles which isn't good for your spine or your head. It's best to position anything you are looking at directly in front of you.

What if you use two monitors? If you use them equally, or even 60/40 my suggestion is that you centre them side by side so you can see each easily. If you are using one more than the other, position the one you use more often, closer to the centre.

Need to share your screen with clients or co-workers? The easiest way to share your monitor and then centre it again for work is to use monitor arms. If this is too expensive, take the time to move the monitor to and from a neutral position. You only have one spine and one neck for a lifetime, so don't risk them for a few minutes of rearranging.

As for the distance between the computer user and the monitor, generally, you want the monitor to be an arms-length away. If you have trouble seeing the monitor, bring it closer, increase the size of your font or consider visiting your optometrist for some computer glasses. I'm going to talk more about vision and computer use in Chapter 9, so I'll save the details for then.

Desk Lamps, Footrests and Document Holders, Oh My!

I thought these unsung heroes of the computer accessories world deserved a mention.

Desk lamps. Working on a computer can be hard on the eyes, so if you don't have enough light for reading at your desk, or if you've turned off overhead lights or closed the curtains to avoid monitor glare, consider a desk lamp. Focus the light where you need it and avoid craning your neck so you can see.

Footrests are the friend of shorter people. If the only way you can get the rest of your body in a neutral posture is to sit so high up that your feet are dangling off the floor, no worries! Use a footrest. Problem solved. They're also a great support for your lower back if you want to work in a standing position.

Document holders are not as common as they used to be, due to the popularity of the paperless office, but if you need to read from a paper document while typing, or if you are reading a large, paper manuscript at your desk, why not use a document holder? Raising the height of whatever you are reading means you don't need to flex your neck and torso forward. Hey, great idea!

Neutral Posture and the Desktop Phone

Ack! Every time I see someone cradling their phone between their shoulder and ear, I cringe! OW! Lots of neck problems are caused by this simple habit. Remember that neutral posture applies to all activities. Obviously cranking your neck to your shoulder for minutes at a time is not good for you, and can cause all sorts of neck and shoulder problems. Instead, hold the phone with your hand, or better yet, use a headset. It may not seem as convenient, but so far modern medicine has not figured out how to replace necks, so you'd better keep yours safe.

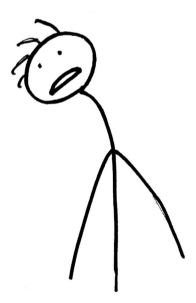

CHAPTER 7:

Neutral Posture and Other Electronic Devices

So far, we've been talking about applying ergonomics principles when working at the home or office computer, but what about other electronic devices? I wanted to focus first on the traditional, desktop computer because it is relatively simple to use it with neutral posture. While it is possible to use other devices in a body-friendly manner, it is often more challenging.

Neutral Posture and the Laptop

Laptops are so very convenient that it's hard to believe they can have a negative side, but a negative side they have. It is simply impossible to use a laptop while in neutral posture. Think about it. The screen and the keyboard are situated so close to each other that you really can't use it without either bending your neck towards the screen or raising your arms to reach the keyboard – or both. Not to mention the effect of resting your wrists on the frame while typing or using the mouse.

> It is impossible to use a laptop while in neutral posture.

Does this mean you can't use a laptop? Of course not! It just means that you need to be smart about it. If you are using a laptop for a short period of time, say 20 or 30 minutes, maybe the awkward posture won't be damaging. Or if you're using your laptop to watch a movie, you're probably not using your hands too much, so it's likely not an issue.

But if you are planning to spend more time on the laptop and will be typing and using the mouse, the safe way to use a laptop is by raising the screen and using an external keyboard and mouse. You can raise your screen either by placing the entire laptop on top of some books or a box, or you can use a notebook stand. What matters is that you are looking directly ahead at the monitor and not leaning forward or down.

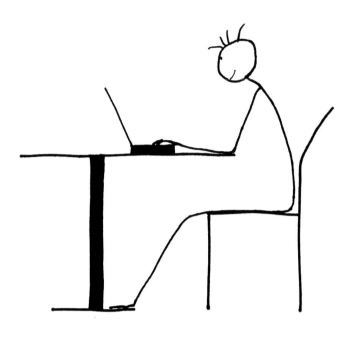

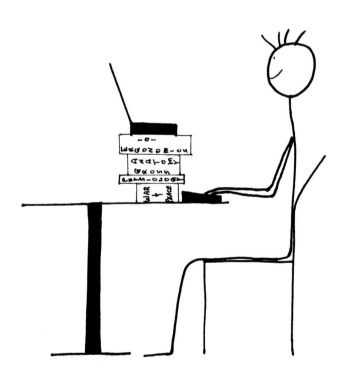

Neutral Posture and the Smartphone

I love, love, love my Smartphone, but darn if these things aren't the culprit for many a sore neck, wrist and thumb. Just look around you, especially in a public place, and look at people's neck posture.

Looking down once in a while is no big deal, but staying in that posture for minutes at a time, or returning frequently to that posture can lead to a really sore neck and sometimes even a headache.

The wrist holding the phone is usually bent in an awkward angle particularly if you are also using the thumb on the same side to text.

Oh the thumb! Thumbs are not designed to type or text rapidly. They are designed to assist the rest of your hand and fingers to grasp items. Opposable thumbs should not be taken for granted – just ask your pet.

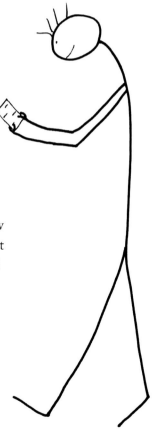

So, how should you use your Smartphone? First, consider using it to call someone instead of texting. I know, I know it's not as convenient, but just putting it out there. When you do text, keep it short and change how you hold the phone. Ideally, hold the phone in the palm of your non-dominant hand so that your wrist is in a neutral position, then type/text using your index finger. That's right, one finger. Don't worry, you'll get used to it and get faster. Plus your thumbs and wrists won't ache and you'll be able to open jars without wincing.

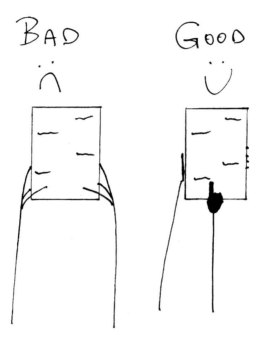

Avoid responding to emails until you are able to use a computer, and try to hold the phone higher when reading or looking at something. Most phones also offer a dictation option, which I've found works really well, as long as you're not in too public a place – that's just embarrassing.

Finally, take breaks. It's easy to lose time when playing a game, or catching up with friends, but try to close your eyes and bring your head up once in a while.

Neutral Posture and the Tablet

Much of what I've said about the laptop and Smartphone can be applied to the tablet. A tablet should be used primarily for looking at information and not writing documents or long posts.

Consider how much heavier a tablet is than a Smartphone. Holding it with one or even both hands requires the wrists to be in an awkward posture which, together with the weight, can easily lead to discomfort in the wrists and forearms.

Further, even if you elevate the tablet and are using an external keyboard to type, you are probably still bending forward to see the screen. Tablets are great for watching stuff, but can lead to problems if used too often for work that should be done on a computer.

To save your neck, rest your hands and the tablet (or Smartphone) on a pillow if you're sitting or lying down. This limits the amount of neck flexion required to see the screen and lightens the load on your wrists and hands.

Neutral Posture While Gaming

This is a toughy. I'm picturing kids (and adults too) sitting on the floor or perched on a chair or sofa while leaning forward, controller buttons and levers being smacked around rapidly by thumbs moving in a blur.

It's pretty tough to sit in a perfect, upright posture and play a game and I've certainly never seen it done. It's also pretty tough to use anything but your thumbs to operate the controls. In my opinion, the best way to prevent repetitive strain injury while gaming is to take frequent breaks (maybe a 5 minute break every 20 to 30 minutes) and to limit time spent gaming. Another great alternative are games that require full body movement rather than hand controls.

If you play games on your computer, you really have a chance to enjoy yourself without injury, assuming you follow good ergonomic principles. Working or gaming at the computer is far more comfortable when using neutral posture. Just take lots of breaks and make sure that you haven't moved your mouse or slouched too far down the chair in the excitement of the game.

CHAPTER 8

Other Risk Factors for Computer Related Injuries

In my opinion, awkward posture is the number one reason why people feel discomfort and even develop Repetitive Strain Injury (RSI) from working at the computer, but there are other factors too:

- contact stress
- static posture
- repetitive motion
- long duration of computer use
- computer/device binging
- lack of physical fitness
- past history of injury or pre-existing condition
- stress

Contact Stress

Simply put, contact stress is when a body part is in contact with a hard surface. If this happens repeatedly and especially with force, it hurts and can cause injury. A perfect example? Leaning on your elbows. Whether you are leaning on your desk or an armrest, "resting" on your elbows can damage the sensitive nerves that run through that valuable joint. If you are experiencing tingling in your little and ring fingers, you might be leaning on your elbow(s) too much.

Another common "resting" place is the underside of your wrist. We've talked about the carpal tunnel a few times now, but the information bears repeating. It pains me to see people typing or using the mouse with their wrists on the desk, or the keyboard, or (argh!) a wrist rest. Let me explain.

Human beings are cleverly designed with weight bearing surfaces. For instance, the bottoms of our feet are quite effective at bearing the weight of our bodies, as are our buttocks when we sit. Our hands also have areas designed for weight-bearing – they are conveniently located in our palms right below the little finger and the thumb. We use these all the time – we rest on the little finger side of our palm when we write and when we are holding utensils (between bites). We use both of these weight bearing pads when we use our upper body to push ourselves out of a chair or off the floor, or when we are doing push-ups.

palm ⟹   designed to bear weight
← designed to make jewelry look good.

The part of our body that we should never use to weight bear is the underside of the wrist. This is because the infamous carpal tunnel is located just under the skin of this part of our wrist. It's a very vulnerable body part because a very important nerve uses this tunnel to go through the wrist and enter the hand. If we put weight on this area we compress the tunnel and all of its contents. When the nerve is compressed, either due to swelling or by putting weight on the tunnel, it typically makes the palm of your hand tingle and can be quite painful. This is commonly referred to as Carpal Tunnel Syndrome.

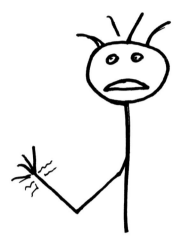

So, how do you avoid Carpal Tunnel Syndrome related to computer use? DON'T REST ON THE UNDERSIDE OF YOUR WRIST. And that includes resting on a gel wrist rest. Palm rests, which provide support to the natural weight bearing surfaces of the palm, are quite comfortable and don't harm your carpal tunnel, but don't confuse them with wrist rests.

Static Posture

Staying in the same position for hours at a time isn't good for you, even if you are in a perfect, textbook, neutral posture. The body is designed to move and needs to move. Unfortunately, many of our jobs dictate that we sit in one place for hours at a time. So what to do?

First of all, make sure that when you are sedentary that you are in a neutral posture (oh come on, you knew I was going to say that). Then, make sure you stand or preferably walk around for at least 5 minutes of every hour that you are sitting and working on the computer. It can be hard to take a break when you're working or to even realize that it's been an hour when you're really focused on your task, but you have an increased risk of injury if you don't. If you already have discomfort, take a break every 30 minutes, or even every 15. As you begin to feel better, you can reduce your break frequency again.

Schedule breaks by using the alarm on your phone or your calendar. You can also purchase break software for your computer and phone. At first these breaks might seem annoying, but it's much better to be slightly annoyed than to have to miss work or miss out on fun at home because you have developed an injury.

Another great way to ensure you move is to drink a lot of water. After you inevitably get up to use the bathroom, get more water. You will feel hydrated and mobile.

Some people are lucky enough to have a sit-stand workstation which allows them to stand while working. This is a great option, but don't forget that your arms and hands need a break too, so you still need to have a 5 minute break at least every hour.

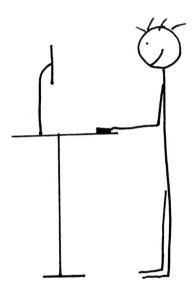

When you are standing make sure you are still using neutral posture in your upper body. Most people don't bring their desks high enough. Remember neutral posture principles apply to both sitting and standing. If you're starting to lean on the desk, or putting most of your weight on one leg, it's time to sit down again.

And if standing up while using the computer is just too weird, then go for a walk. The important thing is to move.

Repetitive Motion

Repeatedly moving the same body part in the same way hour after hour and day after day has consequences. The most common repetitive motion that I've seen with computer use is scrolling. The truth is, many mouse movements are repetitive and the less you use the mouse, the better.

Reducing mouse use can be a real challenge, especially since most of us use the mouse at least twice as much as the keyboard. A great and simple way to reduce mouse use is by learning keyboard shortcuts. Essentially, when you can, use the keyboard rather than the mouse. Often keyboard shortcuts are faster than using the mouse so they are a win/win.

> Keyboard shortcuts are a great way to reduce mouse work and are really efficient once you learn them.

Thinking about getting more active at work by sitting on an exercise ball or using a treadmill as a workstation?

Please don't. It's very difficult to use these devices and maintain a neutral posture while typing and operating the mouse.

Exercise balls are often too low and treadmills tend to result in reaching for computer equipment.

Just move as often as you can and save exercise for the gym where you can focus on your body position and not on your spreadsheet.

I rarely suggest that a person use their non-dominant hand to operate the mouse when their mouse-hand is sore. This is a strategy that does work for a number of people, but in my experience it can lead to discomfort in the non-dominant hand quite quickly, which really leaves you in a bind!

Your non-dominant hand acts as an assistant to your dominant hand; it holds an object steady while the dominant hand manipulates it. When you suddenly ask your non-dominant side to complete a fine motor task, it often over-recruits muscle and force which can lead to injury.

Basically, don't ignore discomfort in one hand by switching sides; the original problem does not go away and you might be adding to your list of aches and pains.

Long Duration of Computer Use

I'm just going to say it. The typical human body is not designed to sit at a computer for more than five consecutive hours per day. More than this, and the body starts to speak to us – sometimes it yells and says bad words. Now, some people can handle more than five hours and some less. Strategies such as taking breaks and using neutral posture can also enable us to work longer on the computer, but there's still no guarantee we won't feel sore.

Numerous people have said to me, "but my job requires me to work for 8 hours a day on the computer." I have two responses to this. First, I understand that technology is progressing at light speed, but it takes much longer for our bodies to evolve, so unless you are a rare and special species of human, you are not capable of doing more computer work than your fellow man.

My second response is that people rarely work on the computer for as long as they think they do. Some of the companies I work for have break software that also tracks computer and specifically mouse usage.

I've noticed that people frequently overestimate the time they work on the computer. I think this is because we don't break up our job tasks into how much time is spent on the computer versus speaking on the phone, attending meetings, using a calculator or chatting with our colleagues. We assume it is all computer work when it actually isn't.

I'm thrilled when people aren't on the computer for as long as they think they are. But when they are, it's time to use some strategies to reduce non-stop computer use.

- Alternate computer and non-computer tasks
- Walk to your colleagues office to talk instead of using email or instant messaging
- Read articles from print rather than on the computer – I know many people crave a paperless office, but it's better for your body and your eyes to step back from the computer and read the old fashioned way. Recycle your paper when you're done.

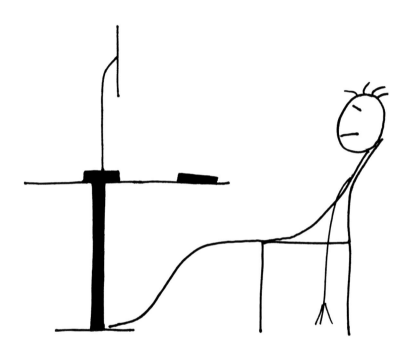

Computer Binging

We all know the saying "everything in moderation," well the same goes for computer use. I've worked with clients who typically don't spend much time on the computer, but have suffered an injury because they chose to spend an entire day organizing their documents into files. Again, spread out your work activities so that you aren't doing all of your computer work on one day.

Lack of Physical Fitness

I know there are more than a few people looking at this header and wondering why a person needs to be fit to complete a sedentary activity.

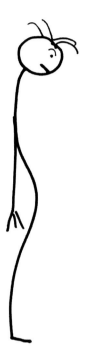

Physical fitness is essential to maintaining neutral posture. We need back and core strength to keep our neck and heads upright and not falling forward. We need to strengthen our rotator cuff muscles so that our shoulder joints are secure and our arms can work properly.

No one needs to be able to run 5 k or spend hours lifting weights to use a computer, but lack of core strength is a real challenge to maintaining good posture.

Pre-existing Injury or Condition

Some people find this hard to believe, but if you live with a condition that affects the normal function of your muscles or skeleton – whether you were born with it or acquired it – you are likely more vulnerable to the risk factors of computer and electronic device use.

For example, if you broke your wrist or hurt you shoulder in a car accident years ago, you may have difficulty achieving neutral posture. If your joint or muscle does not work properly, you might recruit other muscles to help with a movement – muscles that don't normally function in this way and therefore are at increased risk of strain.

The best way to prevent further injury is to ensure you are doing everything you can to attain and maintain full range of motion and strength – usually by completing stretches and strengthening exercises – and of course, by ensuring you are observing ergonomic principles.

Stress

Most people equate stress in the workplace with coping with workloads, schedules and deadlines, but stress from any source has a huge influence on how we feel when participating in activities – including working on the computer.

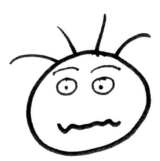

One of the physiological responses of stress is increased muscle tension. Increased muscle tension usually causes muscle soreness and it also makes it hard to have good posture. I have worked with people who have felt sore during the work week, recovered slowly over the weekend and then noticed an increase in physical symptoms on Sunday night while contemplating a return to work on Monday. These symptoms are real and their stimulus is from emotional stress rather than from a physical risk factor.

There are many methods of coping with stress and different things work for different people, but deep breathing exercises seem particularly effective at shutting down our flight or fight response. Any type of body movement is also good for our mood, as is socializing with friends. These are all things you can do at home or in the office, and for any time span that works for you.

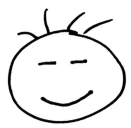

Whatever method you choose, taking the time to be kind to yourself and attending to your mental health will make you a happier, stronger person. We simply cannot underestimate the effect that stress has on our bodies.

Summing It Up

If one or more of these risk factors sound familiar to you, please know that this doesn't guarantee you will feel sore or suffer an injury – but it does increase the likelihood. Be aware of how your body feels and take extra precautions when you recognize these risks.

CHAPTER 9

What You Need to Know About Vision

Many people find themselves in an awkward posture because they have trouble seeing the screen. People using multiple lens or progressive glasses often need to adjust the height of the monitor to be able to read text (we discussed monitor height in Chapter 6: Neutral Posture and Other Office Equipment).

Ideally, you are adjusting the height of the monitor and not the angle of your neck, which of course can lead to neck pain and headaches. But often we make these subtle adjustments without realizing it – sometimes the first notion we have that we've not been sitting correctly is our sore neck. And if you haven't yet read this book, or had an ergonomic evaluation, you might not even know why you are hurting.

It can definitely be challenging to adjust the monitor and the area of the screen you are viewing so that you can consistently see through that elusive window in your glasses. If this is your method of compensating for your vision, be sure to keep your spine and neck in as neutral a posture as possible.

One of my favourite solutions to the "I can't see the screen" problem is…computer glasses!! Most people don't realize that glasses that are designed to compensate for near or far vision are often inadequate for the distance between your eyes and the computer screen. When reading, we typically hold our book or document 16 inches or 41 cm from our eyes. This is also the distance we automatically use for many near vision tasks.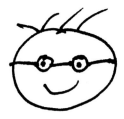

The recommendation for computer screen placement is approximately one arm's length from the user; for me, this is about 28 inches or 71 cm away. Obviously, if I am wearing glasses for reading or other near vision tasks, they are not going to help me read something 28 inches away.

Rather than adopting an awkward posture by leaning forward to read the screen, use computer glasses. Optometrists know all about computer glasses and if you ask them about it, I'm sure they'll be glad to help.

You may wish to continue to use your progressive lenses to read from the monitor, but consider purchasing computer glasses so that you can use the entire lens to see the screen. Often, you can purchase bifocal computer glasses where the majority of the lens is for the screen distance, but a portion of the lower half is designed for reading, which is handy for looking at the keyboard and reading any paper documents you may need to reference.

If you're not ready for computer glasses, or just want to try a few other solutions first, the best and most affordable option is increasing the size of your font.

If you're like me and there are only a few documents that you have trouble reading, try pressing the control button while scrolling the mouse. This will make your document larger or smaller, depending on which direction you scroll, and will make everything much easier to read. The best part? The text remains saved at the font originally used for the document, so that when you send it to someone else, it doesn't show up in the "Wow, this font is enormous!" size and the fact that you can't see everything like you used to, stays your little secret. You're welcome.

Another issue that affects some computer users is sore eyes. If your eyes feel dry, tired and sore after working on the computer, there's a reason for it. Actually, there are several reasons for it.

You don't blink as often when you are working on the computer. We don't know why, but you don't. This is one reason why your eyes feel dry. Another reason is that when you read from a book, you look down and your eyes are partially covered by your eyelid. When you read from a vertical computer screen your eyes are open more widely and so, more of the eye is exposed to air which adds to the dryness. This is such a logical reason for dry eyes, but not something that the average person considers.

Your eyes may also get tired because the lens of the eye is working hard to focus on the words, or picture on the screen. When we read from paper, the lens of the eye focuses on the word and maintains that focus. But when we read from a surface that is backlit, the lens is constantly focusing and re-focusing because the pixels in the screen are not constant. In fact, the centre of each pixel is clear but blurs towards the edges. This mixed image, along with the frequent refreshing of our screens, is not something that we consciously see or notice, but we do notice the fatigue in our eyes.

Solutions for Visual Issues

- Computer glasses

- Increase size of font (control + scroll, or formatting)

- 20/20/20 rule

- Read from paper or E-Reader

- Use "blue" lights that simulate natural sun light

So, aside from increasing the size of our font and wearing computer glasses, what can we do if we experience sore eyes and fatigue from computer use?

One strategy that helps a lot of people is the 20/20/20 rule: every 20 minutes, look at something 20 feet away for 20 seconds. This exercise allows the lens in your eye to relax and also gives you a chance to blink more frequently.

If you are reading a lot from computer monitors, Smart Phones and tablets, you might want to consider reading more often from paper or an e-reader that does not feature a backlit screen.

If you are in an office environment and sit under fluorescent lights all day, ask if you can change the light bulb to a "blue" light, which is designed to simulate natural daylight.

Not everyone experiences visual issues or sore eyes, but keep in mind that, like all computer-related issues, the effects of exposure are cumulative so be aware of the risk and take action if you experience any issues.

CHAPTER 10:

Kids and Ergonomics

So, let's start at the beginning…WAIT! We don't have to, because when it comes to how muscles work in relation to bones and joints, kids have the same body mechanics as the rest of us and we can apply the same ergonomic principles to them as we do to adults.

This is not to say that there are no special considerations for children. Kids are very complex and are constantly developing and growing, which is a great reason for the adults in their lives to ensure children are aware of the importance of good posture from a young age.

> It is not okay for children to use computers, laptops, phones or tablets in an awkward posture.

What I would like parents and teachers to be aware of is this: It is not okay for children to use computers, laptops, phones or tablets in an awkward posture.

Children don't tend to feel discomfort or pain from bad posture as quickly as adults do because their bones and muscles hold more fluid and are more pliable and forgiving. They also tend to move more frequently, which means their awkward postures aren't as static.

However, this doesn't mean that they won't feel discomfort, develop an injury and also develop bad posture habits that they will take with them into adulthood.

There is limited research as to the effects of poor posture and use of electronic devices on children. This is largely due to the speed of technological advances. In fact, technology seems to be growing faster than our kids!

Kids walk funny when they wear our shoes, look silly trying to shave or wear make-up and often need a foot stool to brush their teeth at night, so why do we think they're big enough to use an adult-sized computer workstation?

Also, computers and other electronic devices are accessible to more and more children and at a younger age than ever before. We really don't know the long term effects on children who have awkward posture while using electronic devices because they haven't grown up yet.

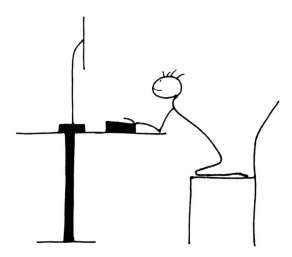

Unfortunately, children as young as five years old are reporting discomfort – mostly in the neck, wrists and arms – from using electronic devices both at home and at school. Some even reported discomfort in their ankles, which puzzled me until I realized they were sitting on their feet in order to reach the keyboard and mouse at an adult-sized workstation.

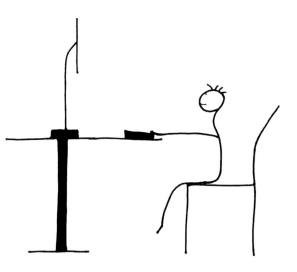

So as adults, what can we do for our children? Adapt the computer workstation, whether at home or at school, to suit the size and needs of the child. All of the neutral posture principles apply:

- Maintain the lumbar curve in the lower back
- Ensure the feet are supported on a stable surface
- The child's bottom should be at the back of the chair and there should be two to four fingers between the back of the knee and the front of the chair (use pillows to adapt chair size)
- Keep the neck, shoulders, arms and hands in neutral posture
- Where possible, provide smaller equipment that is more user friendly for children (see Chapter 14: Ergonomic Solutions for all Budgets)

When your child is playing or doing school work on a computer, ensure they take frequent breaks and try to break up computer work with non-computer activities.

Also, encourage your child to have fun away from the computer, phone and tablet. Growing bodies need to move; a child who plays games on his or her parent's tablet in an awkward position without frequent movement may feel fine in the present, but report discomfort and pain in the future.

Taking the time to set up your child for safe computer use will nurture good habits and prevent future discomfort.

Teach your children how important it is to have good posture when using the computer.

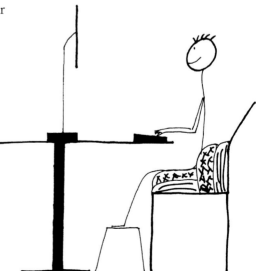

CHAPTER 11

Computer Related Health Risks for Students

When I started working in the field of ergonomics in 2003, it was practically unheard of for someone in their twenties to have computer related discomfort. Unfortunately, it didn't take long for this to change as technology advanced and laptop computers became a mainstay for students at all levels of education.

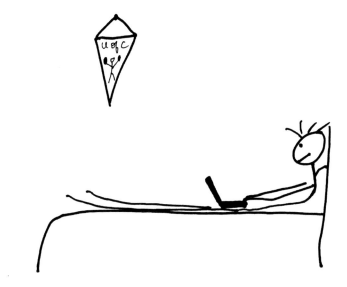

I often provide ergonomic assessments to staff new to the workplace, including university interns. What I have observed is that more and more young adults are arriving to the workforce with discomfort.

One of the most common complaints, and one that gives me great concern, is neck and shoulder pain with tingling and numbness down the arms and hands.

I attribute much of this to countless hours working on homework and university projects on a laptop without an external keyboard and mouse and without raising the height of the monitor.

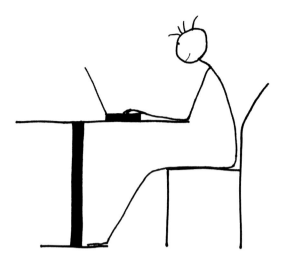

Add to that hours of looking down at the phone while texting and we not only have a generation of people with their heads down, but we potentially have a generation of people who have trouble keeping their neck and head up and in a neutral position.

Most of my young clients are very active and some are athletes.

Despite their efforts to be fit and develop skills in their sport, many are unaware that they are sitting and standing with their neck and heads forward until I show them a picture of themselves.

These young people are so used to maintaining an awkward neck and head posture that it now feels normal to them.

They are usually quite eager to correct their bad habits, especially when they realize how prolonged, awkward posture can affect their function in sports and life in general.

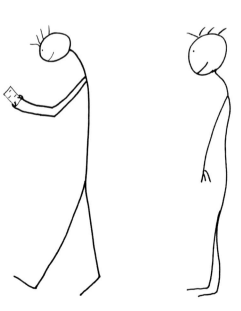

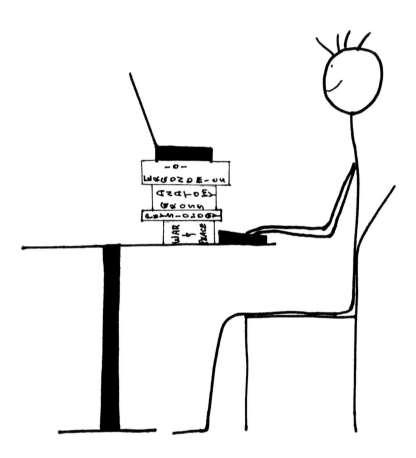

In many cases, the discomfort can be reversed with conscious effort to change postural habits, but for some, the damage may be difficult to treat and even have permanent consequences. These various levels of discomfort and the costs associated with treatment can all be prevented.

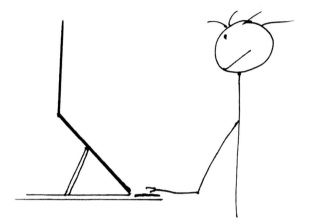

Consider purchasing a notebook stand, external mouse and keyboard for yourself or the students in your home that are using a laptop (see Chapter 14: Ergonomic Solutions for All Budgets).

Advise your child of the importance of setting up a neutral computer workstation for safety. Wouldn't it be great if kids automatically set up their computer for neutral posture just like they automatically put on a seat belt in the car?

Caution young people to reduce texting and to stop using their thumbs to text. I was recently told by a young client that holding your phone with one hand and using the index finger on the other hand to text was a sign of being old. Ouch!

When I recovered, I told the young lady that using neutral posture to text might save her from the pain of tendinitis that is associated with thumb texting. And of course, less texting means less neck bending.

Teach them good ergonomic techniques at a young age and there is a greater chance that they will assume safe behaviours as they approach adulthood.

Older Adults, Special Needs and Ergonomics

All of the ergonomic principles we have discussed also apply to older adults. There are, however, special considerations for people in this age group.

- Muscles and joints possess less fluid and lose strength as we age, and as a result older adults are at higher risk of injury and may take longer to heal than younger people

- Older adults may not be touch typists, which increases the likelihood that they will bend their necks forward to look at the keyboard while they type

- Older adults may have increased difficulty with their vision; some may even have cataracts, glaucoma and macular degeneration

It may not be possible to position older adults into a perfectly neutral posture, especially if they have long-term permanent injuries or health concerns, such as osteoporosis. You are not going to straighten your grandmother's dowager's hump by teaching her ergonomic principles, but a good computer set up will certainly make her more comfortable.

As usual, a good chair is the key to comfort. Many ladies, in particular, require a chair with a shallower seat depth so that they can reach the back of the seat and benefit from the support of the backrest.

I worked with an older woman who felt so much relief from back pain when sitting in her properly fitted computer chair, that she began to use it in her living room when watching television and chatting with visitors.

This is a great example of how good posture affects other activities in our lives; older adults tend to have far less tolerance for awkward postures and a greater appreciation for the relief that neutral posture can bring old pains and injuries.

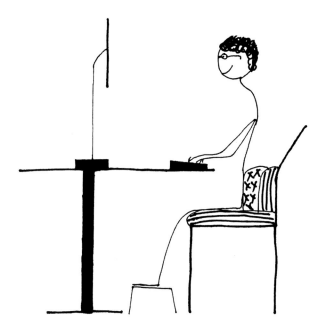

There are also some great keyboards designed for people with visual impairments, regardless of their age. Keyboards may be purchased with larger and/or fewer keys, and a greater contrast of colour between the keys and the rest of the keyboard (yellow keys on a black keyboard seems quite effective).

When it comes to mice, keep it simple. Ensure the wrist is kept in neutral posture and not resting on the desk or table, and don't worry about providing a mouse with numerous buttons unless your older friend or family member is very computer savvy.

Adjust the height of the monitor to accommodate bifocal or progressive lenses – better yet, consider purchasing computer glasses so that you don't need to "search" for the portion of the lens that allows you to read your screen (remember talking about computer glasses in Chapter 9?).

Increase the size of font and desktop icons and remember that it's easier to see objects when there is a greater contrast. Black print on white or yellow background tends to be easiest to read; avoid coloured backgrounds (other than yellow) and text.

Often, as people age, their fine motor skills get worse – the same thing can happen to people of any age who have experienced a neurological condition such as a traumatic brain injury, a stroke, Parkinson's disease or who were born with a condition such as cerebral palsy. People with sore joints from arthritis may also find fine motor tasks, such as typing and using a mouse difficult.

There are numerous aides available for people who are having difficulty physically operating a computer. You can purchase keyboards with fewer and larger keys, mice with larger clicking surfaces and voice recognition software, which can be a good option for some people. There is more information about all of this equipment in Chapter 14: Ergonomic Solutions for All Budgets.

For those individuals with more complex physical challenges, accessibility is often addressed by specialized rehabilitation professionals. Ask your physician for more information.

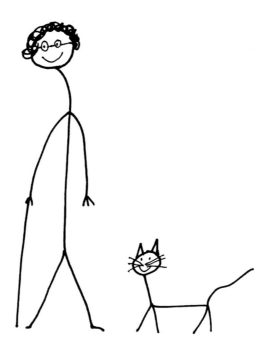

CHAPTER 13

The Fix-It Chart and When to Consult a Health Care Professional

Because the design of the human body is pretty standard – and so is the design of most computers, tablets and other electronic devices – it is often possible to identify what type of ergonomic problem you might have, based simply on the location of your discomfort.

The chart I've created – The Typical Injury, Why It Happens and How to Fix It – focuses on three things:

1. The location of your discomfort or pain

2. What the potential ergonomic cause is

3. How to fix it

I came up with the idea for this chart based on years of experience providing ergonomic assessments for people who complained about pain in the same location and usually as a result of the same ergonomic problem.

It became easy to predict where an individual's pain was located based on looking at his or her workstation, or to guess the nature of the ergonomic problem based on the location of their pain.

The Typical Injury, Why It Happens and How to Fix It

Here it is – the chart with all the answers….okay, maybe not all the answers, but it's certainly a good place to start. The discomfort locations in the chart which I have marked with an asterisk* indicate that the source of the symptoms may be more serious and it is recommended that you see your physician.

Please do not hesitate to see your doctor or another health care professional when you feel discomfort; this chart is intended for use as a guide and a starting place.

You'll notice that the "Fix It" column sometimes includes equipment recommendations. There is a full explanation of all equipment options in Chapter 14: Ergonomic Solutions for All Budgets.

Where it hurts	Possible ergonomic cause	Fix it
*Tingling in hand and fingers	Forward neck posture	• Make sure you're sitting in a neutral position • Adjust monitor so top of screen is at eye height • Use document holder to raise height of reading material • Use closed binder to raise height of reading material • Consider computer glasses
	Contact stress on elbows	• Avoid leaning elbows on desk or armrests • Add double sided tape on armrest to remind you not to lean on elbows • Remove armrests if necessary
	Contact stress on underside of wrist	• Use a vertical mouse or a mouse that will not allow you to rest on the underside of your wrist

Where it hurts	Possible ergonomic cause	Fix it
Top of hand	Too much scrolling	• Reduce mouse use and scrolling by using keyboard shortcuts and arrow keys instead • Keyboard shortcuts for various programs and software are available on the internet • Some keyboards will also allow you to program mouse "hot keys"
Thumb and thumb side of wrist and forearm	Texting	• Use index finger to text; remember, the thumb is not designed to type
	Mouse that uses thumb, such as thumb trackball or joystick	• Switch to a mouse that uses your index and middle finger to click
	Hand is bent towards thumb side of wrist when holding phone/tablet	• Make sure your wrist is in a neutral position • Use a cushion to support the phone/tablet
	Using vertical mouse on surface that is too high	• Raise height of chair or use cushions to sit taller on non-adjustable chair • Lower height adjustable desk so forearms are parallel to floor • Lower work surface by using keyboard tray so that forearms are parallel to floor

Where it hurts	Possible ergonomic cause	Fix it
Little finger side of hand, wrist and forearm	Hand is bent towards little finger side of wrist when texting or holding phone/tablet	• Make sure your wrist is in a neutral position • Use a cushion to support the tablet when using it
	Hand is bent towards little finger side of wrist when typing	• Use split keyboard to attain neutral wrist posture
	Using vertical mouse on surface that is too low	• Lower height of chair or remove cushions if being used to sit taller on non-adjustable chair • Raise height adjustable desk so forearms are parallel to floor • Raise work surface by using keyboard tray so that forearms are parallel to floor
	Using vertical mouse in neutral posture, but for long periods of time	• Alternate between vertical mouse and palm-down mouse daily or weekly
	Contact stress on elbows	• Weight bear only on forearms, not elbows • Avoid leaning elbows on desk or armrests • Add double sided tape on armrest to remind you not to lean on elbows • Remove armrests if necessary

Where it hurts	Possible ergonomic cause	Fix it
Forearm – top	Wrist bent up when typing or using mouse (usually includes resting on the underside of wrist)	• Keep wrist in neutral posture when typing or using mouse • Keep upper arm relaxed at side and elbow bent at 90 degrees (the straighter the elbow, the more likely the wrist will be bent up) • If work surface too low, raise using adjustable desk or keyboard tray • If work surface too low, lower chair, remove cushions on non-adjustable chair
	Too much scrolling	• See "Top of hand"
Forearm – underside	Wrist bent down when typing or using mouse	• Keep wrist in neutral posture when typing or using mouse • If work surface too high, lower using adjustable desk or keyboard tray • If work surface too high, raise seat or add cushions to non-adjustable chair
	Too tight a grip on mouse	• Always use a relaxed grip on mouse

Where it hurts	Possible ergonomic cause	Fix it
Elbow	Often an extension of forearm discomfort	• See "Forearm" recommendations
	Contact stress on elbows	• Avoid leaning elbows on desk or armrests • Add double sided tape on armrest to remind you not to lean on elbows • Remove armrests
Upper arm – front	Reaching forward to use keyboard or mouse (often accompanied by sore shoulder blade)	• Sit closer to the work surface • Make sure you can access mouse and keyboard while keeping elbows at 90 degrees • Mouse and keyboard should be next to each other and not on different work surfaces (e.g. one higher than the other) • Maintain neutral posture by keeping shoulder/arm relaxed at side while working

Where it hurts	Possible ergonomic cause	Fix it
Upper arm – side	Reaching to side for mouse (often accompanied by sore shoulder blade)	• Bring mouse closer to keyboard • Use narrower keyboard
	Sitting with hand on armrest and elbow out to side	• Move armrests closer to body e.g. directly under shoulders • Put tape on armrest as a reminder to keep hand off of armrest • Remove armrests and do not lean on desk or table • Consider exercises to strengthen core
	Sitting with arm "resting" on armrest that is too far away from body (leaning away from neutral position)	• Move armrests closer to body e.g. directly under shoulders • Put tape on armrest as a reminder not to use it • Remove armrests and do not lean on desk or table • Consider exercises to strengthen core
	Sitting with arm slung over backrest	• Put tape on backrest as a reminder not to rest arm on backrest • Consider exercises to strengthen core

Where it hurts	Possible ergonomic cause	Fix it
Upper arm – back and shoulder	Reaching for keyboard or mouse	• Sit closer to the work surface • Make sure you can access mouse and keyboard while keeping elbows at 90 degrees • Mouse and keyboard should be next to each other and not on different work surfaces (e.g. one higher than the other) • Maintain neutral posture by keeping shoulder/arm relaxed at side while working
	Posture of upper back and neck is forward and rounded	• Make sure you're sitting in a neutral position • Adjust monitor so top of screen is eye height • Raise height of laptop and use external keyboard and mouse • Use document holder to raise height of reading material • Use closed binder to raise height of reading material • Consider exercises to strengthen core • Consider computer glasses • Reduce texting or raise height of phone/tablet
Neck and top of shoulders	Shoulders are raised and too close to ears	• Relax shoulders into neutral position • Lower armrests • Remove armrests

85

Where it hurts	Possible ergonomic cause	Fix it
Neck – side	Cradling phone between ear and shoulder	• Hold phone with hand • Use phone headset
	Monitor off to side, not centred	• Centre monitor • If using two monitors and using both equally, centre both • If using two monitors and using unequally (70:30 or greater), position most used monitor closer to centre
Neck – back	Bending head down to see paper documents, books	• Use document holder to raise height of reading material • Use closed binder to raise height of reading material
	Texting, playing games on phone	• Hold phone higher when texting, playing games • Take frequent breaks and/or reduce texting and playing games on phone
Neck and between shoulder blades (middle back)	Leaning forward to see screen	• Consider computer glasses • Increase size of font
	Leaning forward while typing or using mouse (often occurs when resting forearms on work surface)	• Make sure sitting with buttocks at very back of chair • Adjust chair or cushions to properly support lower and upper back if using non-adjustable chair • Take frequent breaks
	Seat too deep	• Reduce seat depth on adjustable chair or add cushions to non-adjustable chair

Where it hurts	Possible ergonomic cause	Fix it
Inside shoulder blade of mouse arm	Reaching to side for mouse	• Bring mouse closer to keyboard • Use narrower keyboard
	Sitting with arm "resting" on armrest that is too far away from body (leaning away from neutral position)	• Move armrests closer to body e.g. directly under shoulders • Put tape on armrest as a reminder not to use it • Remove armrests and do not lean on desk or table • Consider exercises to strengthen core
Lower back	Lumbar support not in proper place	• Adjust lumbar support • Add cushion or rolled up towel to non-adjustable chair
	Not moving enough	• Take breaks • Stand/walk throughout day • Break up computer work with non-computer work tasks
	Seat depth or height not appropriate	• Adjust seat of chair • Add or remove cushions from chair to achieve correct height • Use footrest if feet not firmly resting on ground

Where it hurts	Possible ergonomic cause	Fix it
Buttocks/ Back of thighs	Seat depth too shallow and/or seat height too low	• Raise height of chair or add cushions to non-adjustable chair • Increase seat depth • Consider purchase of adjustable chair with greater seat depth and height
Hips	Not moving enough	• Schedule breaks on computer or with co-workers • Make sure chair set up correctly
	Crossing legs while working	
Ankles	Sitting on feet (usually smaller people or children)	• Adjust chair and workstation for size of user • Use footrest

When to Consult a Health Care Professional

Despite the insight that this chart can provide, my hope is that you will never hesitate to get a professional ergonomic assessment – it really can improve your quality of life by reducing pain and avoiding the costs of treatments that may only provide temporary relief.

If you get your evaluation from an occupational therapist like me, you might even be able to use your benefits plan to pay for it. If your benefits plan doesn't cover occupational therapy, consider asking them to add this service, or use funds from your Health Spending Account.

> If your benefits plan doesn't cover occupational therapy, contact your service provider and request that it be added.

Regardless of how you pay, the cost of prevention is minor compared to the cost of treatment, time away from work, not to mention the cost to your health and quality of life.

When you request a professional, ergonomic assessment, recommendations may include equipment, behavioural changes regarding posture and breaks, and often stretches and strengthening exercises. I've included a short list of stretches for you in Chapter 15: Simple Exercises for Relief and Prevention.

It's best to ask for help before your discomfort transitions to actual pain, but if your discomfort has escalated to the point where you need some treatment for pain relief you may need additional professional help. This is usually when I recommend my physiotherapist friend or you may wish to see a chiropractor. Treatment programs should relieve pain AND prepare your muscles and joints for stretching and strengthening exercises.

Regardless of what type of health professional you choose to see for treatment, keep in mind that you will ultimately feel better, maintain your health and prevent a reoccurence by being diligent about doing your exercises (and following ergonomic principles, of course). I've never known someone to experience permanent resolution of discomfort and injury by simply paying someone to provide a treatment while you lie passively on a table.

There are times when you definitely should consult with a health care professional for an ergonomic evaluation and for physical treatment.

- If your pain is severe
- If you are experiencing tingling in your extremities
- If you have been diagnosed with a condition which is chronic and/or progressive

Long-term solutions rarely happen by simply paying someone to provide a treatment while you lie passively on a table.

As an example for this last bullet point, consider an individual with rheumatoid arthritis. As a registered occupational therapist with years of experience, I am aware of the typical progression of this joint disease, body postures to avoid and how to maintain function and prevent the aggravation of symptoms. Working with someone who has the knowledge of both ergonomics and human pathology is definitely beneficial.

CHAPTER 14

Ergonomic Solutions for All Budgets

My goal when providing ergonomic recommendations is to provide solutions that fit an individual's or a corporation's budget, environment and purpose.

Above all, the answer to "How To Fix It" must be practical.

I've organized this chapter into equipment sections and have attempted to provide you with a few options and tips for making computer work/ play safe for you and your family.

I've purposefully avoided providing brand names, and have instead suggested equipment features you should aim for. I've listed the equipment items in order of **most ideal to least ideal** and have tried to include prices where possible. Obviously, prices will vary depending on where you live, so take these with a grain of salt.

Chairs *(pages 94-96)*

It kills me when people own great equipment, but don't have it set up properly. I've consulted for businesses who have spent $900 on very expensive chairs, but $0 on educating their staff on how to use them. As a result, by the time I got there, tall people were sitting on small chairs, small people were sitting in large chairs and the adjustable features were covered in dust bunnies. The moral of this story? If you choose to purchase a good chair, learn how to use it or hire someone to show you how.

Desks *(pages 97-100)*

The distinguishing feature between a table and desk that are designed for computer work, is that a desk may be in an "L" shape and feature a corner unit for computer placement, whereas a table is a simple, rectangular-shaped work area.

Here are a few more tips:

- Tables tends to be more affordable than desks
- Desks that are designed with a corner unit that is not curved possess some challenges
  - The chair armrests may prevent the chair (and you) from getting close enough to the desk to access the keyboard and mouse in neutral posture
  - Solve this issue with corner maker "filler" that can be purchased from most furniture stores, or if you're handy, make your own
  - Solve this issue by working on the straight side of the desk, or purchase a desk with a curved corner unit; the purchase of a table or one-sided desk may be a better and more affordable solution especially for a home office

Keyboard Trays and Mounts *(pages 101-102)*

If you do not have an adjustable height desk/table, or if it doesn't go low or high enough, a keyboard tray with an adjustable mount may be the answer.

Please Note: Many keyboard trays come with a wrist rest attached—remove these prior to use. Remember that resting on the inside of your wrist means you are compressing your carpal tunnel.

Monitor Arms and Risers *(pages 103-104)*

You can use stack books under your laptop or monitor to raise the height, but it's always nice to have something in place that's designed for this purpose.

Document Holders *(page 105)*

Raising the height of something you're reading or referring to while using the computer is a great neck-saver. These range from the very simple, to holders that have adjustable height and angle. Remember to place the document holder directly in front of you, not to the side.

Footrests *(page 106)*

A footrest of some kind is essential for shorter people whose feet don't reach the floor when the rest of the body is set up in a neutral position. If your feet aren't firmly on the floor, your body is not being properly supported.

Laptop Accessories *(page 107)*

If you want to use a laptop, you will NOT be able to achieve neutral posture and prevent injury if you don't have an external keyboard, mouse and a stand to raise the height of the laptop.

Keyboards *(pages 108-111)* and Mice *(pages 112-114)*

There are a large variety of keyboards and mice available and for the most part, one is not necessarily better than another—it's really dependent on the size of the person using the item and what kind of work/play is being done.

You'll notice that I haven't included the cost for any keyboards or mice on the chart—there are simply too many choices. There are some fantastic devices available in stores and online, and a higher price doesn't always translate to a better product.

CHAIRS	Pros	Cons
Adjustable Chair with: • Adjustable seat height • Adjustable seat depth • Adjustable lumbar support • Backrest tilt feature • Adjustable armrest height • Adjustable lateral movement of armrests	• This chair can place anyone in an ideal, neutral posture • Ideal for a workstation that is shared • Chairs can usually be ordered with different sized seats as well e.g. larger seat depth and height for tall people and shallower seat depth for shorter people and children • Can also be purchased with wider seat and back rest for people over 300 lbs • Armrests can be adjusted for height and can be moved closer to body for smaller people	• Estimated cost between $700 to $1000
Adjustable Chair with: • Adjustable seat height • Adjustable lumbar support • Adjustable armrest height	• This chair is usually a good choice for people between 5'4" and 5'11" • May also be available in different seat depths for shorter and taller people • Estimated cost between $300 to $600	• May require use of cushions to adapt seat depth for smaller people • May not be as comfortable for people over 6' • Armrests cannot be adjusted closer to body, so will not support arms of smaller people in a neutral position

CHAIRS	Pros	Cons
Kitchen Chair	• Readily available in most households • You already have it! Which makes it better than the height only adjustable chair, since you have to add props, like pillows, to both of them	• Will require use of pillows for lumbar support for all people • Will require pillows to increase height and reduce seat depth for smaller people • Seat may be too shallow for tall people • Footrests will be required for smaller people
Adjustable Chair with: • Adjustable seat height • Non-adjustable lumbar support	• This chair will work well for a small group of people who are exactly the right height and build for the chair • Appropriate for short-term use e.g. one hour at a time • Estimated cost between $100 and $300	• Chair will not be comfortable for the majority of people for long-term use • Pillows or lumbar support cushions will be required to provide lumbar support • Is not cost effective since it may require purchase of cushions, etc. to compensate for simplicity of chair • Will not support neutral posture for the majority of people, so additional costs for health care professional assessment and treatment are likely

CHAIRS	Pros	Cons
Lumbar Support Cushions and Backrests	• Can be an affordable way to adapt a kitchen chair, or a less adjustable office chair (if you have already purchased one) • Estimated cost between $8 and $400	• May need to re-adjust frequently • Full-sized back rest cushions may have a lumbar support that is not adjustable • Is a poor substitute for a better chair • The cost of a poorly adjustable chair plus a lumbar support cushion may be similar to the cost of a more adjustable chair
Towels and Pillows	• You already have it! • You can adjust the size of lumbar support by choosing a different sized pillow or towel, or rolling the towel more tightly or loosely	• May need to re-adjust frequently • May not provide adequate support

DESKS/TABLES	Pros	Cons
Height adjustable desk/ table –electronic	• Many people think the best feature of adjustable workstations is that you can stand to work BUT the very best feature is that you can adjust the seated height of the workstation to any size of person – this is priceless • Almost effortless to adjust height, making it more likely that you'll adjust when necessary • Some feature programmable buttons so you can save the workstation height for each user, or program the heights for sit or stand for a single user • Estimated cost $600 and up (and when I say up, think $6000)	• Although they are getting more affordable, most are still out of the price range of the average home office user • I have heard of people buying electronic tables for as little as $600, but you must look for these deals – don't hesitate to visit office furniture stores and ask if you can purchase a floor model • Also, be aware that lower priced models will likely be less stable • If you are under 5'2" or over 6'2", make sure that the range of height will accommodate your size – not all workstations have the same range of adjustability

DESKS/TABLES	Pros	Cons
Height adjustable desk/table – crank	• Similar to electronic workstation, but must use a hand crank to adjust • Much more affordable than the electronic version • Estimated cost $300 and up	• Adjustment feature is not used as often because of the perceived effort of using the hand crank – especially if using the workstation for only a short period • As for the electronic version, understand the range of adjustment before you buy and that lower priced models will likely be less stable
Leg-height adjustable desk/table	• Can be a great choice for a single user, or same-sized people • Height is adjusted when setting up the desk to suit the needs of the users • Estimated cost $200 and up	• Not good for use with different sized people • Although height can be adjusted after initial set up, most have to be dismantled in order to do this, so it is rarely readjusted • Usually not adjustable for standing height

DESKS/TABLES	Pros	Cons
Non-adjustable desk/table	• The most affordable option, assuming you are not too tall or too small • Can be used safely with smaller people if have height adjustable chair and a foot rest • Usually lower than kitchen table so a better option • Can be found for under $100	• Some users, especially taller people, will not be comfortable even with extra props • Props, such as footrests, keyboard trays and chair height adjustment take time, so effort must be made to sit in a neutral posture for some people
Kitchen table	• You already have it! • With firm pillows and footrests, it is possible to set up work in neutral posture	• Usually too tall for neutral computer work unless you are over 6'3" • Adapting for use with neutral posture takes time and effort • Can be a tough place to work because of location

DESKS/TABLES	Pros	Cons
Height adjustable riser	• Neat device that can be used on any surface to raise your working height • Enables people to work in standing • Many varieties, so price can range from $70 to $500	• Intended to allow people to work in standing, not to adjust seated workstation height • May not rise high enough for tall people • Make sure monitor height is changing as well as keyboard and mouse height • Affordable, but if buying a new desk, consider if buying a nicer desk/table is comparable in price to buying a cheaper workstation plus a riser
Upside-down cardboard box	• You probably have one, or can find one for free • If you've got the right height and size of box, it's a great option	• May not be the right height • May not be strong enough • Looks messy

KEYBOARD TRAYS AND MOUNTS	Pros	Cons
25 to 27" wide keyboard tray	• Wide enough to easily hold keyboard and mouse • For price, see "Adjustable mounting arm for keyboard tray"	• May be too wide for some corner unit desks
<25" wide keyboard tray	• Narrower trays will fit into most work spaces • For price, see "Adjustable mounting arm for keyboard tray"	• May not be wide enough to hold both keyboard and mouse • If mouse or keyboard is on a different work surface, neutral posture will not be achieved = you will spend money on sore shoulder
Adjustable mounting arm for keyboard tray	• Allows for a wide variety of keyboard tray heights and angles • Can be used with a non-adjustable desk or table to make the workstation the right height for a wide variety of people • Can be added to adjustable desk/table that does not have a large enough range for very tall or small people • Estimated cost between $200 and $400, including tray	• Definitely more expensive than the non-adjustable version

KEYBOARD TRAYS AND MOUNTS	Pros	Cons
Non-adjustable mounting arm and keyboard tray	• Does not adjust for different heights or angles • A great prop if your desk/table surface is an inch or two too high • Estimated cost between $40 and $200; tray width will vary	• You must be the perfect sitting height to use this in a neutral posture • Tend to work well for people 5'4" to 5'8" tall
Built-in keyboard tray	• A good option if it fits your body size and shape • Estimated at under $100 (with desk); tray width will vary	• Like the office chair with the built-in, non-adjustable lumbar support, this is only a good option is you are exactly the right size for the desk and tray.

MONITOR HEIGHT ADJUSTERS	Pros	Cons
Adjustable monitor stand	• Most monitors come with a stand and many of them are height adjustable • Look for a wider range of adjustability if you are tall or small • Estimated price – usually included with price of monitor	• May not have a large enough range
Monitor arm	• Allow for a wide range of mobility • Handy when you want to share your screen • Allows for easy adjustment for multiple monitor use • Estimated price between $100 and $800 – depending on adjustability and number of monitors	• The more mobility is featured, the higher the cost • Most require a hole to be made in your desk/table for mounting • Keep in mind that what you get is what you pay for – cheaper monitor arms may not stay in place or support heavier monitors

MONITOR HEIGHT ADJUSTERS	Pros	Cons
Monitor riser	• Cheap and easy to find in most box stores • Can buy stackable risers • Estimated cost $10 to $50	• Only adjusts in height • Takes time to move riser and monitor
Books/boxes	• Usually free and readily available	• May not be strong enough to hold monitor • May be unbalanced • May not be correct height

DOCUMENT HOLDERS	Pros	Cons
Angle and height adjustable document holder	• The adjustability means documents can be placed directly in front of the monitor and centred to the user • Height adjustability means the screen will never be obstructed by the holder • Estimated cost $75 to $300	• All the adjustability can make it less stable and not as good for books or large documents
Angle adjustable document holder	• The adjustability means documents can be placed directly in front of the monitor and centred to the user • Tend to be sturdy and good for use with books and larger documents • Estimated cost $75 to $300	• No angle adjustability
Closed binder	• Almost every office or household has one • Handy for computer use or for reading paper documents – the larger, the better	• Not adjustable
Non-adjustable document holder	• Can purchase for as little as $10	• Not adjustable, so if you use it to reference documents while working on the computer, you will likely have an awkward neck position

FOOTRESTS	Pros	Cons
Adjustable footrest	• May have 2 or 3 adjustable heights for different users and for different ankle positions • Great to use when standing at desk/table to relieve pressure on lower back • Estimated cost $60	• The more adjustable an item is, the more expensive it is
Non-adjustable footrest	• Cheap and easy to find in most box stores • Great to use when standing at desk/table to relieve pressure on lower back • Estimated cost $20	• Not as adjustable
Foot Stool	• May already be available in household • Strong enough for use as long as correct height • Estimated cost $10 to $50	• May not be correct height
Books/boxes	• You already have it!	• May not be strong enough • May be unbalanced • May not be correct height

LAPTOP ACCESSORIES	Pros	Cons
Notebook stand • Lightweight, portable stands that hold your laptop upright so that the screen may be positioned for neutral posture	• Promotes neutral posture and a safe method of using a laptop • Easy to take with you on a trip or to the library if you're a student • Estimated cost is $80	• Usually has to be ordered online
Books/boxes	• Usually free and readily available • Promotes neutral posture and a safe method of using a laptop	• May be unbalanced • Not convenient to take with you
Light weight keyboard and mouse	• Reduce risk of awkward posture and contact stress that occurs when using laptop keyboard and mouse • Estimated cost of mini keyboard is $60 to $100 • Estimated cost of cordless mouse is $20	• Must take with you
Laptop bags • Carry your laptop and accessories conveniently	• Backpacks are great when you are not around pavement and/or using public transit • Estimated cost $50 to $150 • Roller bags are best used for airport travel and/or when around pavement • Estimated cost is $100 to $300	• An added expense, but a necessity for most laptop owners

KEYBOARDS	Pros	Cons
Wide (19" or more)	• May have larger keys which are easier to locate • Generous spacing between keypad and number pad • Generally easier to find in local stores • Allow most men and broader people to access the keyboard and mouse with neutral posture	• Too wide for some men and most women and children to access the mouse without reaching beyond neutral posture • Some keyboards that are advertised as "ergonomic" are far too wide for safe mouse use and are misleading
Narrow (16" or less)	• Perfect width for most women and children • Can be used safely by most men, although the keyboard is often perceived as too small	• Usually has to be ordered online
With number pad	• The number pad is essential for people working with a lot of spreadsheets or in finance • Narrower keyboards are available with and without number pads	• May make keyboard too wide for safe mouse access

KEYBOARDS	Pros	Cons
Without number pad	• Good for people who don't need number pad • Takes up less room on work surface • Can be as narrow as 11" • 11" keyboard can be used successfully with most children and is light for travel	• Usually has to be ordered online • Not practical for people working with spreadsheets, or in finance
Number pad on left	• Allows right handed people to use mouse with right hand and number pad with left • Keyboard is centred to body with number pad and mouse on either side, like bookends	• Usually has to be ordered online • Can be very difficult to get used to, as home keys are shifted slightly to right
Split	• Great for people who tend to type with their wrists bent towards their little finger • Often allows neutral typing posture for people with arthritis, or people with large girth	• Usually has to be ordered online • Usually does not include a number pad • Can be very difficult to get used to, as home keys are shifted slightly to either side • Splitting the keyboard can increase the width, compromising mouse position

KEYBOARDS	Pros	Cons
Separate number pads	• Great for people who need a number pad but want the flexibility of moving it to the right or left of the keyboard, or removing it from the workspace entirely • A good option to accompany split	• Usually has to be ordered online • If placed on same side as mouse, can result in excessive reaching for mouse in a non-neutral posture
For the visually impaired • Fewer keys • Higher contrast colors (yellow background with black letters) • Larger print • Braille	• Greatly improves computer access for people with visual impairment including people with retinopathy, and older adults	• Usually has to be ordered online (but remarkably easy to find)

KEYBOARDS	Pros	Cons
For those with poor motor skills • Isolates important keys so it is easier to press them without accidentally pressing others	• Greatly improves computer access for people with compromised motor function	• Usually has to be ordered online
For children • Usually have fewer keys so easier for small hands with developing coordination to use • Very colourful	• Narrow keyboard makes it more likely that the child will use the mouse in a neutral posture • Particularly good for children with motor control issues (please note that these children are often seen by occupational therapists who will likely recommend equipment for them)	• Usually has to be ordered online • Usually more expensive than a very narrow, 11" keyboard which might be a good choice for a child

MICE	Pros	Cons
Traditional palm down	• Most people are very used to this type of mouse • Usually easy to buy locally	• This design often results in people resting on the underside of the wrist – which may lead to carpal tunnel problems!
Traditional palm down with palm rest	• Combining a traditional palm down mouse with a palm rest makes it a very safe, neutral-friendly mouse • Palm rest can be paired with any palm down mouse, but it works best with a cordless mouse • Good choice for traveling and for students	• Make sure you are resting on the fleshy parts of your palm (see Chapter 8, page 45) and not on your wrist
Vertical • Hand rests on small finger side of palm while operating the mouse • There are a variety of angles of vertical mouse, ranging from thumb side of hand facing the ceiling to almost palm down mouse position	• Positions the forearm in neutral posture • Mimics our natural hand position used for eating, writing • Can be very comfortable • Eliminates risk of resting on underside of wrist	• Usually has to be ordered online • Can be difficult to get used to • Wrist must be in neutral posture (not bent towards thumb or little finger side of hand) or will result in discomfort

MICE	Pros	Cons
Left-handed (non-dominant hand) • Many people assume using your "other" hand to operate the mouse when your dominant hand is sore is a good solution – this is not always the case • Using the mouse is a fine motor activity and the non-dominant hand isn't trained for fine motor activity – it is a helper for the dominant hand • Often, the non-dominant hand will over-recruit muscles when using the mouse and will develop an injury faster than the dominant hand	• Many mice are available for right or left handed use • Switching between right and left handed mouse work is a good strategy for people who are ambidextrous • Often people who are left handed are able to use their right hand to mouse easily	• Usually has to be ordered online • May result in discomfort to non-dominant hand

MICE	Pros	Cons
Trackball – hand	• Often works well for people who want to use more shoulder and hand movement and less wrist and finger movement	• Usually has to be ordered online
Trackball – thumb	• Relies on the thumb to operate most mouse controls, which allows fingers and sometimes wrist to rest	• Usually has to be ordered online • High risk of overusing thumbs and not recommended
Joystick	• Relies on the thumb to operate most mouse controls which allows fingers and sometimes wrist to rest	• Usually has to be ordered online • High risk of overusing thumbs and not recommended
Pen and tablet	• May reduce scrolling movement and allow index finger to rest • If very flat, so that it simulates pen and paper, can be a good option	• Usually has to be ordered online • Most tablets are not flat like paper and require the "pen" hand to rest on a hard edge when accessing the tablet • May result in contact stress and injury to the wrist

CHAPTER 15

Simple Stretches for Relief and Prevention

Sometimes a simple stretch can make a big difference in how you feel. I've included a few stretches that are a great daily practice, even if you don't have discomfort or pain – and they can all be done in your office!

Whole Body Awareness

Standing in Neutral Posture

Remember this guy? Once in a while we need to remind ourselves what standing up in a tall, neutral posture, feels like.

Instructions:

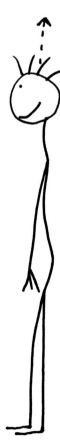

- Stand up straight, putting equal weight on both feet and relax your arms at your side

- Imagine a string coming from the top of your head and gently pulling your head towards the ceiling

- Take a moment to notice how your neck feels – is it positioned differently now? What about your shoulders? How does your lower back feel?

- Think about how your body feels in neutral posture and try to maintain this posture as you sit at your workstation, complete household tasks, hobbies or crafts or play games

Neck

All stretches should begin by first attaining neutral posture, but starting in neutral posture is even more important for neck stretches.

I recommend doing most stretches in standing since it is more challenging to attain neutral posture in a seated position.

How long should you hold a stretch? Good question! There are a lot of different opinions, but 30 seconds seem to be a fairly common response.

If you can't or don't want to hold a stretch for that long, please stretch even if it's for a shorter period.

Side Neck Stretch

Instructions:

- Stand in neutral posture with shoulders relaxed and arms hanging at sides
- Slowly bend your neck to the side bringing your ear towards the shoulder – don't force it, just allow your neck to gently bend as far as is comfortable
- Make sure your shoulder remains relaxed and does not come up towards the ear
- Hold and bring neck back to neutral position
- Repeat with the other side
- Complete 3 times each side

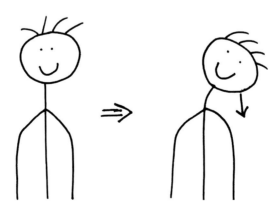

Side Angle Neck Stretch

Instructions:

- Stand in a neutral posture with shoulders relaxed and arms hanging at sides

- Turn you head to the right and stop when you are about half way between the neutral position and your right shoulder

- Very slowly, bend you neck down and hold

- Return the neck to the neutral posture by slowly reversing your movements: bring your neck up and rotate it back to neutral position

- Repeat with the other side

- Complete 3 times each side

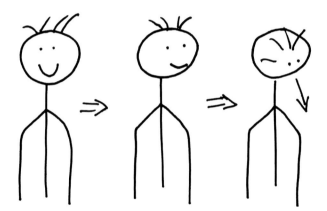

Shoulders and Neck

There are many people who really don't know how to relax their shoulders. Improving your awareness of what a relaxed, neutral shoulder posture feels like is a great skill to have.

Instructions:

- Stand in a neutral posture with shoulders relaxed and arms hanging at sides

- Shrug your shoulders up towards your ears and hold for 5 seconds

- Release your shoulders into a relaxed position

- This relaxed posture is where your shoulders should be when you're standing, working at the computer, talking with friends – basically all the time!

You can use the exercise below while seated at a computer chair to make sure your armrests are set at the correct height.

Tense shoulder posture can be a sign of stress.

Recognizing that you have tense shoulders means you can do something about it – like this stretch.

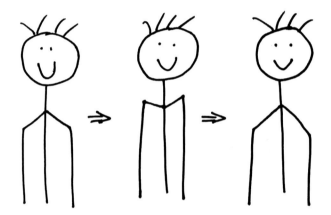

Instructions:

- Sit in a neutral posture with your upper arms at your sides and your hands in your lap – a perfect resting posture.

- Now leave one hand in your lap and put the opposite arm on the armrest.

- Do you feel a difference in the height of your shoulders? If your armrests are up too high, it should feel obvious and if it doesn't just take a picture.

- Your armrests should support your neutral posture, not force your arm and shoulder into a muscle-fatiguing position.

Chest

Instructions:

- Stand in neutral posture, next to a doorframe
- With your elbow bent, lift your arm out to the side so the elbow is at shoulder height
- Place your elbow and forearm on the doorframe
- Slowly lean forward and hold
- Return to neutral posture and repeat with the other side
- Complete 3 times each side

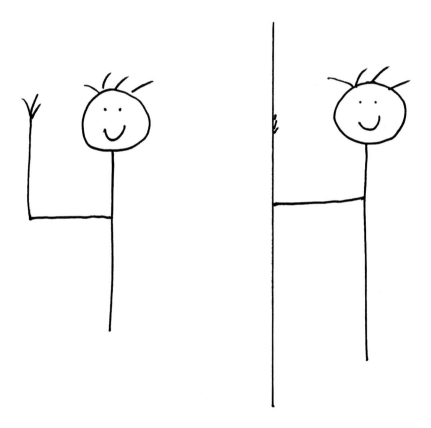

Upper Arm

Instructions:

- Stand in neutral posture, next to a doorframe
- Keeping your elbow straight, lift your arm out to the side – raise it only as high as you feel comfortable
- Gently grasp the door frame with your hand
- Slowly lean forward and hold
- Return to neutral posture and repeat with the other side
- Complete 3 times each side

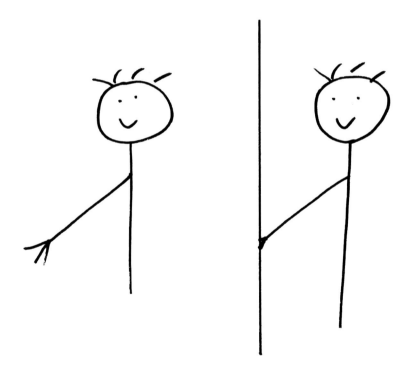

Top of Forearms

Instructions:

- Standing or sitting in a neutral posture, bring your right arm in front of your body with the elbow straight and palm facing the ground

- Using the opposite hand, gently push down the right hand, and hold

- Release and repeat with the other side

- Complete 3 times each side

Underside of Forearms

Instructions:

- Standing or sitting in a neutral posture, bring your right arm in front of your body with the elbow straight and palm facing the ceiling

- Using the opposite hand, gently push down the right palm (make sure you are placing the opposite hand on the palm and not on the fingers), and hold

- Release and repeat with the other side

- Complete 3 times each side

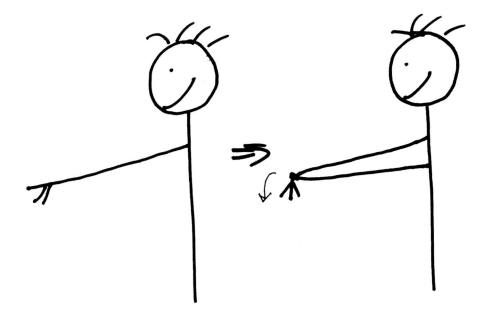

Hands

Instructions:

- Standing or sitting in a neutral posture, hold both hands in front of body and spread your fingers and thumb as wide as possible (jazz hands – silly grin optional)
- Relax and make a gentle fist
- Complete 3 times

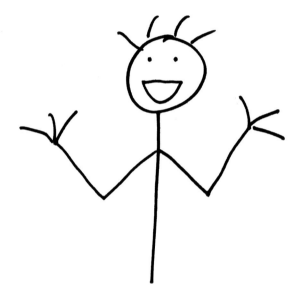

Instructions:

- Standing or sitting in a neutral posture, hold both hands in front of body
- Slowly touch the tip of the thumb to each finger tip
- Repeat, increasing speed each time
- Complete 3 times

Mid-Back

Instructions:

- Stand in a neutral posture with shoulders relaxed and arms hanging at your sides
- Position feet slightly wider than hip width apart, with knees slightly bent
- Bring both arms forward as if you are hugging a large barrel, allowing your fingers to touch
- Your back will naturally bend to accommodate this position
- Hold and return to neutral posture
- Complete 3 times

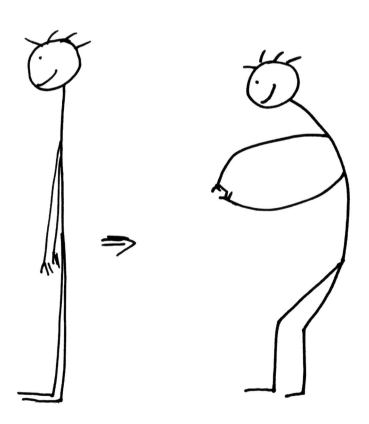

Lower Back/Pelvis

This stretch is similar to the yoga cat and cow poses, but is completed in standing. This is a great stretch if you've been sitting for long periods of time.

Instructions:

- Stand with legs wide apart and knees bent at about 45 degrees

- Place hands on top of thighs and keep back straight

- Slowly curl your pelvis under so that your lower back is bent and your bottom is tucked inward

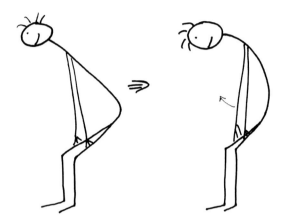

- Your middle and upper back will naturally bend to accommodate this position

- Hold and return to the starting position

- Pause and keeping hands on knees, slowly arch your pelvis and lower back in the opposite direction as the first bend, pushing your bottom out

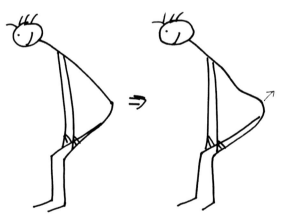

- Hold and return to starting position with straight back

- Complete 3 times

Front of Hips

The muscles in the front of your hip (your hip flexors) can get really tight if you sit for much of the day. This is a great stretch to reduce muscle tightness and can reduce lower back strain as well.

Instructions:
- Stand in a neutral posture with shoulders relaxed and arms hanging at your sides
- Keeping the upper body upright, take a large step forward with the right foot and hold with the knee bent
- Keep the left foot on the ground in its original position – make sure you maintain an upright posture
- You should feel a stretch in the front of your hip
- Hold and bring right leg back to starting position
- Complete 3 times on each side

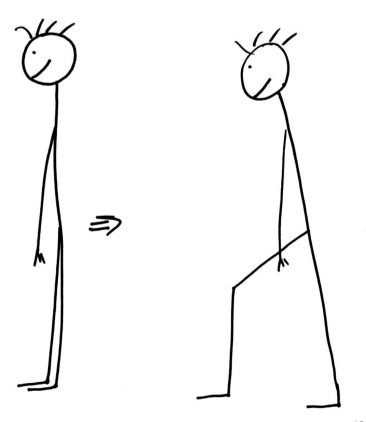

Front of Thighs

Instructions:

- Stand in a neutral posture with shoulders relaxed and arms hanging at your sides

- Keeping your hips in a neutral posture, bring your right heel towards your right buttock

- Grasp your right foot (or if you can't reach it, your pant leg) with your right hand and hold

- Do not allow right leg to come out to side, but keep right thigh next to the left

- You may use the wall or a chair to assist with balance as needed

- Hold and release to neutral posture

- Repeat with the other side

- Complete 3 times each side

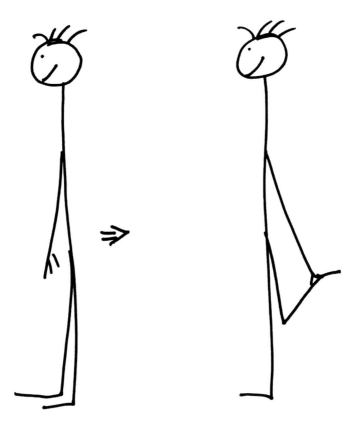

Back of Thighs

Instructions:

- Stand in a neutral posture with shoulders relaxed and arms hanging at your sides

- Bring right foot forward, heel to the ground, toes up and knee straight

- Left foot will remain at starting position, but left knee will bend

- Keeping the back straight, bend at the hips, place your hands gently on the left thigh and hold

- Return to the starting position and repeat with the other side

- Complete 3 times each side

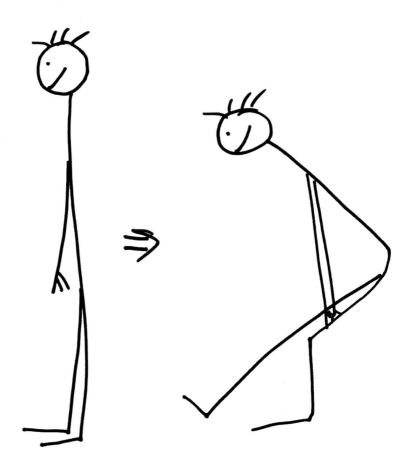

Calves and Ankles

Instructions:

- Stand in a neutral posture with shoulders relaxed and arms hanging at your sides

- Slowly raise both heels so you are standing on your toes and return to starting position

- Complete 3 times

Instructions:

- Stand or sit in a neutral posture

- Lift one foot off the ground and rotate the ankle first clockwise and then counterclockwise

- Return the foot to the ground and repeat with the other foot

- Complete 3 times each side

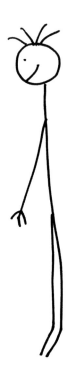

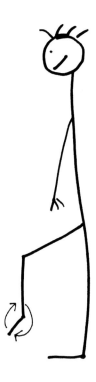

Conclusion: Putting it all together

Well you made it to the end of the book! Thanks for staying with me!

I've always enjoyed providing ergonomic assessments and educating people on health prevention and the importance of good posture, so I'm thrilled to be able to share my knowledge and experience in this book.

In case you forget, here are a few key points to remember:

- There are **health risks** associated with poor posture – for people of all ages
- **Money** spent on passive treatments alone is money wasted – you must identify the source of the problem and be an active participant in the solution
- **Pain** is often preventable and in many cases can be eliminated, not simply tolerated
- **Neutral posture** is how our bodies are designed to move, and if we work or play in an awkward posture, eventually something might break
- Take the time to make sure your computer workstation is **set up properly** – use pillows and boxes if you don't have the funds to buy adjustable equipment

It's been a pleasure sharing with you. I hope you find the information helpful for you and your friends and family, at work and at home.

Thanks and take care!

Your occupational therapist,

Irma

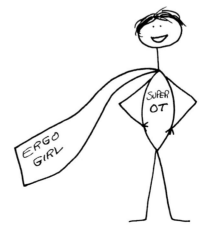

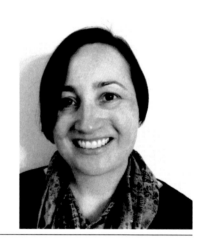

ABOUT THE AUTHOR

Irma became an occupational therapist (O.T.) in 1995 and finds working with clients and promoting health extremely rewarding. When she's not trying to "save the world" with occupational therapy, Irma enjoys an active lifestyle and also has a creative side. Irma lives in Calgary with her wonderful husband, and her demanding cat. She loves spending time with them and the rest of her extended family and friends.

Irma is passionate about ergonomics and health promotion and is available for speaking engagements for your group or business. You can contact her at **www.janzenotservices.ca**.